Illnesses

Dr Teresa Kilgour

Pub
in a   n

Some of the photographs in this book have been reproduced courtesy of the
Science Photo Library

© Family Doctor Publications 2007

Family Doctor Publications, PO Box 4664, Poole BH15 1NN

BMA Consulting Medical Editor: Dr Michael Peters

ISBN-13: 978 1 903474 14 3
ISBN-10: 1 903474 14 0

Contents

About the author

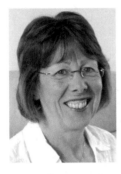

Dr Teresa Kilgour is an Associate Specialist in Community Paediatrics. She is a graduate of St Andrew's and Manchester Universities and recently obtained a Masters Degree in Child Health from Leeds University. She works for City Hospitals Sunderland, providing paediatric support to the Sure Start Children's Centres in the area.

Introduction

Parents have a demanding job!

As a parent of three sons and a daughter, all born within six years of each other, and with a career in community paediatrics, I agree with the comment that being a parent is one of the most difficult jobs in the world.

There is no instruction manual and no one teaches you how to do it. Parents must be multi-skilled, needing to cook, clean, wash, iron, play, read stories, teach, manage accounts, referee fights and quarrels, be fancy dress makers, taxi drivers and the rest, and all of this without pay!

As if this were not hard enough, children often become ill, which makes the task of parenting even more difficult because it is always an anxious time when this happens. Caring for an ill child can be very demanding and requires patience and understanding. Parents are often faced with three problems:

1 Is the child really ill?

2 When do they seek medical advice?

3 Children react in different ways to illness.

How do parents know when a child is ill?

The first problem is to recognise when children are really ill. It can be very confusing; one minute they may seem really unwell, feeling hot, listless and generally unhappy, and the next they are up and running around, and there appears to be nothing wrong with them.

When to seek advice

The second problem is to know exactly what to do. Should I call the doctor? Should I take him or her to the nearest accident and emergency department (known as A&E)? Should I just wait and see how things go?

The answer is: if you are in any doubt, you should always err on the side of caution and contact your family doctor. This is particularly important for babies and younger children who cannot describe their symptoms and tell you exactly how they feel.

All children react differently

The third problem is that symptoms of illness can vary from child to child and they can also react differently to being unwell – for example, some children like to be cuddled when they are unwell, whereas others just want to be left alone. Some children become flushed, whereas others have an unusual pallor (look very pale).

Children may not want to eat or drink, may be coughing or breathless, may have a rash or be drowsy or listless, have sniffles or maybe they have no specific symptoms.

Parents may not be able to diagnose the specific problem but they instinctively know when there is something wrong. It is worth remembering that most bouts of illness pass quickly and leave a child better able to resist the next attack.

Organisation of the book

This book is divided into chapters, the first giving a general description of infections and fever, and the next six describing illnesses that affect particular systems of the body. Each of these six chapters starts with a description of the anatomy of the relevant body system. The eighth chapter explores the concept that 'prevention is better than cure'.

Throughout the book I have explained medical terms that you may have heard when visiting the hospital or your doctor in an attempt to demystify medical language. Some medical terms sound complicated but may have quite simple meanings.

I hope by reading this book that you may gain an understanding of some of the more common childhood illnesses, which, in turn, may help to alleviate some of the anxiety surrounding them.

KEY POINTS

- Caring for a poorly child can be very demanding and requires patience and understanding

- Recognising when a child is ill is not always obvious

- Most bouts of illness pass quickly, but if you are in doubt seek medical help

General infections and fever

Causes of childhood illnesses

Most childhood illnesses are caused by viral infections and a smaller number by bacterial infections. These organisms can enter the body in a variety of ways but most commonly are breathed in or swallowed. They can also enter through a break in the skin or are brought in by another organism such as a flea or mosquito when it bites.

Viruses

These are the smallest known infective organisms. They consist of nothing more than a piece of genetic material, surrounded by a protein coat. They can multiply only inside a living host cell, but once they are inside they multiply very rapidly.

Viruses may affect cells in different ways, for example:

- They may kill the cell.

- They may remain in the cell for some time and have no immediate effect, but they can become active at a later date.

The body's defence mechanisms have to work to destroy viruses; with a few exceptions antibiotics do not kill them. Some of the most common viral infections in children are those affecting the nose, throat and lungs – the area of the body referred to as 'the upper respiratory tract' (see page 50).

Many different virus groups can affect us and within each group there are also different types (strains) of the same virus. For example, the virus that is the main cause of the common cold has many different forms, each of which needs purpose-built body defences to overcome it.

Each time that you are infected you become immune to that particular strain and therefore gradually build up resistance to viruses. This is why an average child may catch eight or more colds a year whereas adults catch fewer.

Bacteria

These are also single-cell organisms, but they are larger than viruses although still very small. They come in a variety of shapes, which account for the names of the main groups – bacilli are rod shaped, cocci are spherical and spirillae are curved. Not all bacteria cause disease and some live within our bodies without causing any harm and, in some cases, do good. For example, bacteria in the gut help to break down products of digestion and they can also prevent the growth of harmful bacteria.

The differences between bacteria and viruses

Both viruses and bacteria are microscopic organisms that can enter the body cells.

1. Viruses

Viruses are minute organisms. They are parasitic in that they are dependent on nutrients inside cells to survive and reproduce. A virus is very simple, consisting of a strand of genetic material covered by protein.

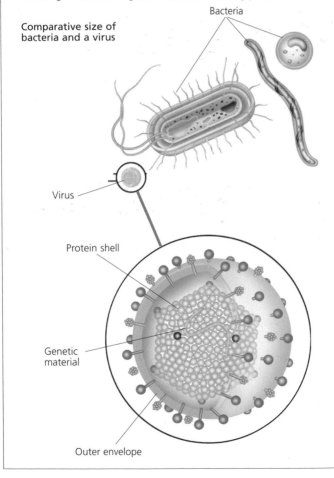

Comparative size of bacteria and a virus

Bacteria

Virus

Protein shell

Genetic material

Outer envelope

The differences between bacteria and viruses (contd)

2. Bacteria

There are three principal forms of bacteria – spherical, rod shaped and curved. Most bacilli and spiral forms have independent movement from the flagellum – a whip-like structure. If bacteria produce disease they are called pathogenic.

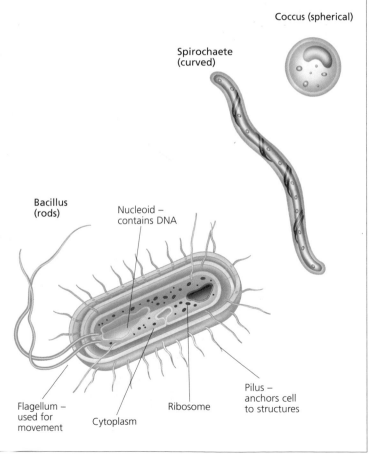

Coccus (spherical)

Spirochaete (curved)

Bacillus (rods)

Nucleoid – contains DNA

Flagellum – used for movement

Cytoplasm

Ribosome

Pilus – anchors cell to structures

Bacteria cause illness in one of two ways:

1 They enter the cell through the cell membrane and multiply rapidly inside. The newly formed bacteria rupture the cell membrane and spread to other cells in the body.
2 They produce poisonous substances called toxins that either kill the cells directly or affect their function.

Bacterial infections often cause more serious illness than viral infections but antibiotics are effective in destroying them.

Antibiotics
A group of medicines called antibiotics kill bacteria by entering the cell and interfering with the mechanism that forms their walls, which then causes them to disintegrate. Viruses have a simpler structure against which antibiotics are ineffective.

The overuse of antibiotics can actually do more harm than good because bacteria can build up a resistance to them. This can result in antibiotics becoming less effective against some of them – for example, the MRSA (meticillin-resistant *Staphyloccocus aureus*) bacterium – which is why it is important that antibiotics are used only when they are really needed.

Defence mechanisms
The body has its own defence mechanisms to deal with invading organisms. The main components of the body's immune system are the white (actually colourless) blood cells.

How antibiotics work

Some antibiotics break down the bacterium's cell wall so destroying it. Others are absorbed into the bacterium where they destroy it by disturbing its essential functions such as protein synthesis.

1. Breakdown of cell wall

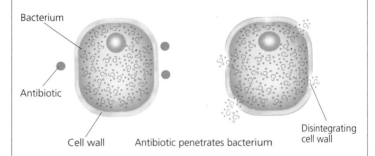

Bacterium

Antibiotic

Cell wall

Antibiotic penetrates bacterium

Disintegrating cell wall

2. Interruption of function

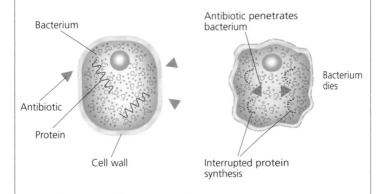

Bacterium

Antibiotic

Protein

Cell wall

Antibiotic penetrates bacterium

Bacterium dies

Interrupted protein synthesis

There are five different types of these blood cells, each with different functions:

1 Neutrophils: engulf harmful organisms and then kill them.

2 Eosinophils: also engulf organisms and are important when larger organisms infect the body.

3 Lymphocytes: provide early defence by producing protein antibodies that match up with individual bacteria. After the first infection with a particular organism, the lymphocyte recognises if it invades again and it is destroyed as soon as it enters. This explains why viral infections such as measles usually result in lifelong immunity or resistance to re-infection from the same virus.

4 Monocytes have a similar role to neutrophils but they live for much longer. They also help the lymphocyte response.

5 Basophils do not actually engulf bacteria but these cells have a major role in allergic responses.

Fever

Raised temperature, or fever, is the body's way of fighting infection. The blood temperature rises in an attempt to kill invading organisms, such as bacteria. Fever is one of the most common reasons for a parent seeking medical advice. The normal body temperature is 36 to 37°C (96.8 to 98.6°F) and a fever is described as a temperature greater than 37.7°C (100°F).

The body's temperature varies slightly during the course of the day so, for example, it is a little lower in the morning and a little higher at night. It also fluctuates, particularly in children, as they run around, play or become over-excited, or are perhaps over-dressed.

A raised temperature on its own is not a cause for concern and is the body's natural way of fighting an infection (see below).

Measuring a child's temperature

Taking a child's temperature is not as easy as it may seem. Children do not like sitting still and will wriggle and squirm to stop you trying to take it. There are a variety of different thermometers available to measure a child's temperature.

Glass mercury thermometers

Glass mercury thermometers were widely used in the past but are now considered too dangerous to use because of concerns about the glass breaking and consequent exposure to mercury, which is extremely toxic. A glass mercury thermometer is also difficult to read; there is a knack to visualising the column of mercury.

Digital thermometers

Newer thermometers mostly have a digital (number) display – either centigrade or Farenheit – making them easy to read. These are placed either in the armpit or under the tongue for an older child.

Ear or aural thermometers

The best combination of accuracy and comfort for the child is found in aural, or ear, thermometers, which have a disposable tip that is inserted into the external ear canal; the reading takes a few seconds.

Strip/forehead thermometers

Strip thermometers, which are held against a child's forehead, are not as accurate as other types but are cheap, safe and easy to use. They can confirm a parent's suspicion that his or her child has a fever.

Treatment for fever

There is currently some debate about whether a fever should be treated (reduced) because it is one of the body's natural defence mechanisms. However, if a child is uncomfortable it is probably best to reduce the fever. This is achieved in the following way:

- Dress in cool, light clothing: children should not be wrapped up if they have a raised temperature. A vest, nappy or pants and a light sheet are all that is necessary.

- Keep the room well ventilated and not too warm; there is no evidence to suggest that fanning the child is helpful.

- Give your child plenty of cool drinks: try ice-lollies and ice-pops if your child does not want to drink.

- Give the recommended dose of paracetamol or ibuprofen (unless your child has asthma – see page 60) for your child's age. It does not matter which one you give, so it is best to use the one with which you are familiar and that you find is most effective. The temperature should fall by 1°C (2°F) one to two hours after the medication has been given. It may not fall back to a normal level.

- Tepid sponging is no longer recommended.

Important
- Do not give aspirin to children under 16 years of age because it is now known to be associated with a rare, but very serious, illness known as Reye's syndrome.

Measuring a child's temperature

Parents usually sense when their child has a fever – the forehead and body will be unusually warm. There are a number of ways to measure a child's temperature.

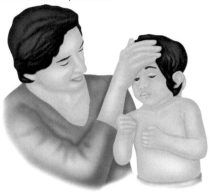

1. Digital thermometer
Placed under the tongue or armpit

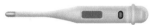

2. Strip/forehead thermometer
Held against the child's foehead

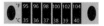

3. Ear sensor
The tip is placed inside the ear – very quick and accurate

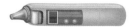

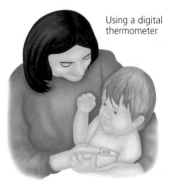

Using a digital thermometer

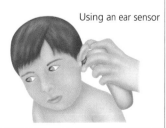

Using an ear sensor

- Do not put a child in a cool bath as this will cause the surface blood vessels to narrow and the body's core temperature may then rise even further.

- Do not give ibuprofen to a child with asthma because it may worsen the symptoms.

When to seek medical help

If the above measures do not work and the child has any of the following symptoms, medical help must be sought:

- The temperature is greater than 39°C (102°F).

- The temperature returns after going away for 24 hours.

- If the child has a stiff neck (child can't put her chin to her chest).

- If the child is crying inconsolably.

- If there are any signs of dehydration, for example, severe thirst, passing much less urine than usual, a sunken fontanelle (the soft spot on top of a baby's head), or very dry lips and mouth.

- If the child is unwilling to lie down.

- If there is any difficulty breathing.

- If the child is floppy.

- If the child develops a purple/red rash anywhere on the body.

- If the child is unusually drowsy.

- If there is any confusion.

Febrile seizures

Also known as fever fits, febrile seizures are convulsions brought on by a raised temperature in very young children – they usually occur in children aged

How to give medicine to small children

Most medicines are supplied with a measurement tool – for example, a spoon or syringe.

From a syringe
A sterilised medicine syringe can be useful for very young children. Immerse the plunger in the medicine and draw up the required volume. Try squirting the medicine inside your child's cheek to avoid choking.

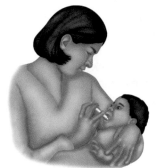

Using a dropper
Measure the dose into a spoon and then fill the dropper.

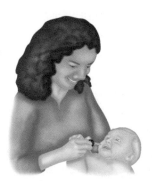

Using a spoon
This can be messy, but even young babies can be persuaded to take medicine from a spoon.

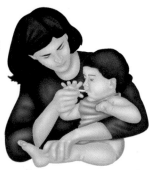

between six months and five years, and affect about one in every 25 children. The seizure seems to occur as a response to the rapid increase in temperature that results in an abnormal burst of electrical activity in a child's brain cells. They are particularly common in toddlers.

Any illness that causes a high temperature can trigger a seizure but the most common infections to do so are those affecting the upper respiratory tract, for example, ear or throat infections. Seizures occur most frequently at the beginning of the illness.

Recognising a febrile seizure

During a febrile seizure a child usually loses consciousness. The child's arms and then the legs go stiff; this may be followed by shaking of the limbs. The child's eyes may roll upward. Breathing may become shallow and irregular, which may result in his or her lips turning a bluish colour. Most febrile seizures last a minute or two. Once the seizure has stopped the child may sleep deeply for a few hours.

Although seizures are extremely frightening for parents, most are not serious and the child will make a complete recovery. However, further seizures may occur if the child has another feverish illness; about 30 per cent of children are affected in this way.

There are a number of factors that seem to make it more likely that a child will have recurrent seizures:

- If the first seizure occurs before a child is 15 months old.
- If any other members of the family have had febrile seizures either as children or as adults.
- If the child has frequent febrile illnesses.

Seizures and epilepsy

Parents are understandably anxious that a child who has had one or more seizures may later develop epilepsy. The risk is very small; only 1 per cent develop epilepsy later in life, compared with a chance of 0.4 per cent that epilepsy will develop in a child who has never had a febrile seizure. Most children outgrow this tendency and it is very rare for children aged over six years to have further febrile seizures.

Treatment for febrile seizures

It is very important for parents to stay calm and keep first aid to a minimum:

- Don't restrain the child during the seizure.

- Don't place anything inside the mouth.

- Do remove any objects from the mouth that might obstruct breathing.

- Do move any hard or sharp objects out of the way of the child to prevent injury.

- To prevent choking, the child should be placed on his or her side once the seizure has stopped.

- If a seizure has not stopped after five minutes, emergency medical help should be summoned immediately.

- Once the seizure has ended, attempts should be made to bring a child's temperature down.

- If a seizure has not stopped WITHIN five minutes, emergency medical help should be summoned (CALL AN AMBULANCE).

After a seizure: lay the child on his or her side, with the upper arm and leg bent at the elbow and knee, and tilt the head back slightly. This will keep the air passages open and prevent choking.

Preventing further febrile seizures

It is commonly advised to try to reduce a child's temperature when he or she has an illness, but there is no evidence that this will decrease the risk of further seizures. However, a child will certainly feel more comfortable if his or her temperature is lowered and it seems sensible to treat it (see page 12).

Children who are prone to febrile seizures do not necessarily need to be admitted to hospital every time. They may need to be admitted only if there are signs of a serious underlying infection, such as meningitis.

KEY POINTS

■ Most childhood illnesses are caused by viral infections

■ In general antibiotics do not kill viruses

■ Bacterial infections often cause more serious illness than viral infections but antibiotics are effective in destroying them

■ A normal temperature lies between 36 and 37°C (96.8 and 98.6°F) and a fever is described as a temperature greater than 37.7°C (100°F)

■ The treatment of a fever involves simple practical measures

■ Febrile seizures occur in some children when they have a temperature and may recur

The eyes, ears, nose and throat

Common conditions

Conjunctivitis, sore throats, earache, runny noses and intermittent hearing loss are all extremely common conditions in children. Knowledge of the structure of the eyes, ears, nose and throat, and their close anatomical connections, is important in helping you to understand these symptoms and how and why one infection can quickly lead to another.

The eyes: conjunctivitis

This condition is an inflammation of the conjunctiva, the thin membrane that lines and protects the surface of the eye and the inside of the eyelids. It usually starts quite suddenly, often in one eye, and then quickly spreads to both, because the child may rub the affected eye and touch the other one.

Conjunctivitis can be caused by an infection with bacteria or viruses or it can result from an allergic reaction or a reaction to an irritant. Bacterial

Anatomy of the ear, nose and throat

The ear, nose and throat are all interconnected, so an infection in one part can quickly transmit to another area.

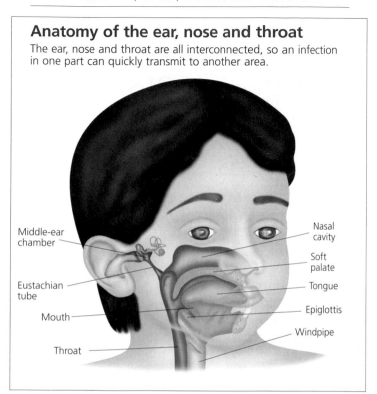

Middle-ear chamber

Eustachian tube

Mouth

Throat

Nasal cavity

Soft palate

Tongue

Epiglottis

Windpipe

conjunctivitis is usually caused by *Staphylococcus* species, *Streptococcus pneumoniae* or *Haemophilus influenzae*. Viral conjunctivitis is commonly associated with upper respiratory tract infections and is usually caused by the adenovirus. Allergic conjunctivitis is a frequent symptom of hay fever.

Symptoms of conjunctivitis

- Redness of the eye: blood vessels over the white of the eye become very prominent
- Swelling of the eyelids

- Discomfort: the eye is itchy and often described by adults as burning or gritty
- Stickiness around the eyelids: a discharge develops from the eye that is particularly problematic in the morning when the eyelids can be stuck together; the discharge can be thick and yellow or clear and watery
- Occasionally children complain that the light hurts their eyes (photophobia).

Treatment for conjunctivitis

Conjunctivitis caused by bacteria or viruses is extremely infectious. You should wash your hands thoroughly after touching the eye in order to prevent it spreading. Give your child separate towels and face cloths, and change the pillowcase daily. Keep your child away from nursery or school during the acute stage of the infection; this is when the eyes are obviously red and sore.

For allergic conjunctivitis

Ease the symptoms with anti-allergy drops. As there are many different types on the market, it is best to obtain advice from your pharmacist. If the eye becomes increasingly red or painful medical advice must be sought.

For viral conjunctivitis

There is generally no treatment for viral conjunctivitis unless it is caused by the herpes virus, when antiviral drops can be used. It may help to bathe the eyes with cooled boiled water, but great care must be taken not to spread the infection. Before and after treating your eyes thoroughly wash your hands and nails.

The structure of the eye

Each eye is roughly spherical, but only a small part is visible. The eyes are protected in the skull by the eye sockets.

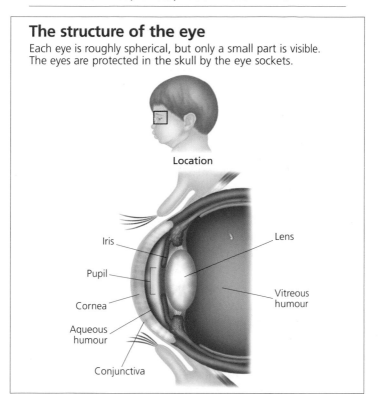

Location

Iris

Pupil

Cornea

Aqueous humour

Conjunctiva

Lens

Vitreous humour

For bacterial conjunctivitis

This must be treated with antibiotic drops or ointment. Although infective conjunctivitis is self-limiting and does not cause any serious harm, the use of antibiotic drops increases the rate of improvement. If the symptoms do not clear with treatment, a swab will be taken and sent to the laboratory for analysis, so that the correct antibiotic can be prescribed.

Conjunctivitis in the newborn

When a newborn baby develops conjunctivitis, this has to be treated immediately to avoid long-term damage to the eye. It can be the result of an infection from the mother's vagina that is transmitted to the baby's eyes during birth. This form of conjunctivitis is usually caused by sexually transmitted infections (STIs) such as infection with *Chlamydia* species or gonorrhoea.

The ears

Your ears are the organs of hearing and balance. An ear has three functional parts: the external ear directs sound waves to the eardrum; a middle ear, which relays the vibrations of the eardrum to the internal ear; and the inner ear itself. It is the inner ear that translates the vibrations into nerve impulses that the brain can interpret; the inner ear also contains the organ of balance.

Ear infections are very common in children. They can affect any part of the ear, and the signs and symptoms vary according to where the infection is situated.

The external ear

This consists of an auricle – the visible part of the ear – and an external ear canal. This tube is about four centimetres (two inches) long and lined with skin that contains many wax-secreting glands. It ends at the eardrum, a translucent oval membrane that separates the external ear from the middle ear.

The middle ear

This part of the ear is filled with air and contains a chain of three tiny bones linked to the eardrum: the malleus (hammer), incus (anvil) and stapes (stirrup); the function of these is to transmit vibrations from the eardrum to the inner ear through a structure called the oval window.

The structure of the ear

The ear is a remarkable part of the body sensing sound and balance. It is divided into three parts: the outer, middle and inner ears.

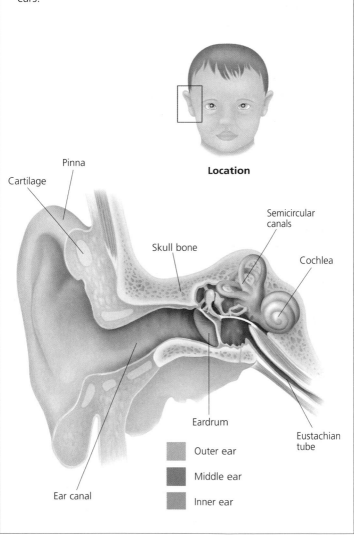

Location

Pinna

Cartilage

Semicircular canals

Cochlea

Skull bone

Eardrum

Eustachian tube

Ear canal

Outer ear

Middle ear

Inner ear

The outer ear

The outer ear is a canal about four centimetres (two inches) long, comprising an outer third that is lined with hairs and an inner two-thirds that have a bony wall lined with a thin layer of skin.

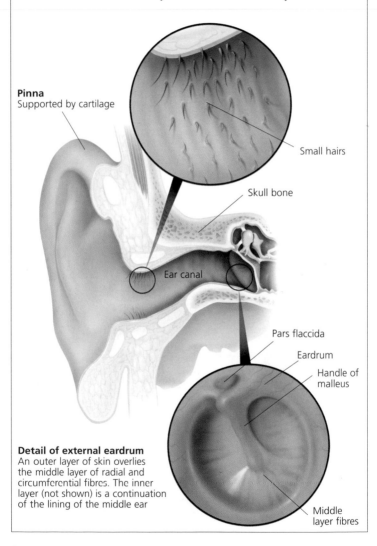

Pinna
Supported by cartilage

Small hairs

Skull bone

Ear canal

Pars flaccida

Eardrum

Handle of malleus

Detail of external eardrum
An outer layer of skin overlies the middle layer of radial and circumferential fibres. The inner layer (not shown) is a continuation of the lining of the middle ear

Middle layer fibres

The middle ear

The middle ear is an air-filled space that holds three small bones (ossicles) which connect and transmit vibration from the eardrum to the inner ear.

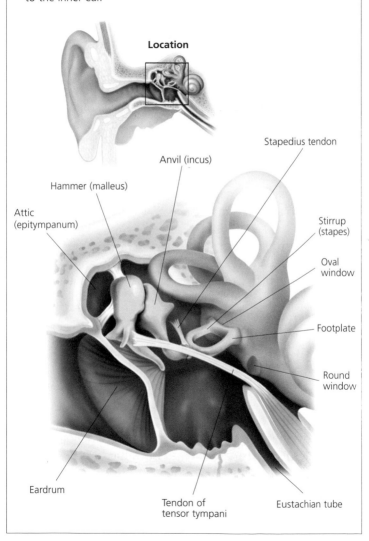

Location

Stapedius tendon

Anvil (incus)

Hammer (malleus)

Attic (epitympanum)

Stirrup (stapes)

Oval window

Footplate

Round window

Eardrum

Tendon of tensor tympani

Eustachian tube

Eustachian tube

This connects the middle ear to the back of the nose and throat. It allows air to circulate in the middle ear and can provide a pathway for infection to pass from the throat to the middle ear.

The inner ear

The inner ear has two main parts: the cochlea and semicircular canals. The cochlea is a coiled bony tube, divided into three channels, one of which contains the receptor for hearing. This receptor converts the vibrations from the middle ear into electrical signals. Nerves carry these signals to the brain, where they are interpreted.

The semicircular canals are filled with fluid and detect movement and balance.

Examining the ear

Your doctor will examine a child's ear with an instrument commonly known as an otoscope, although it is sometimes called an auroscope. This provides magnification and a bright light source so that a good view can be obtained of the external canal and eardrum. The doctor will pull the ear upwards and backwards to straighten the external canal in order to obtain a clear view of the eardrum.

Otitis externa

This is the term used to describe an inflammation of the external ear canal, whereas otitis media is an inflammation of the middle ear. (Otitis is a term derived from the Latin word for the ear.) The inflammation of otitis externa is often but not always accompanied by infection. It can complicate eczema and is common in

The inner ear

The balance portions of the inner ear can detect acceleration of the head in any direction, whether in a straight line or twisting and turning to the inner ear.

Semicircular canals

The three semicircular canals lie at right angles to each other. The canals are fluid filled and each contains a sensory organ called a crista, which is capped by the cupula

When the head moves, the fluid in the canals displaces the cupula, stimulating the nerves in the crista

Location

Vestibule

There are two fluid-filled chambers each containing a sensory organ called a macula. When the head moves, the gelatinous membrane of the macula is displaced, stimulating the nerve

Vestibular nerve

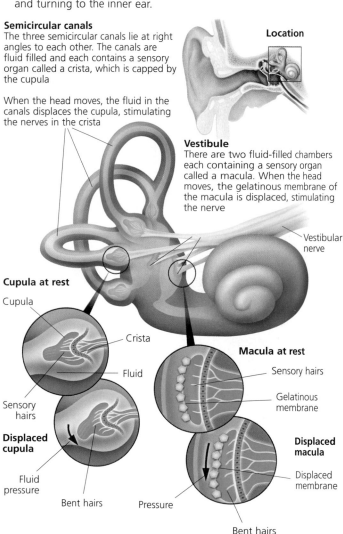

Cupula at rest

Cupula

Crista

Fluid

Sensory hairs

Displaced cupula

Fluid pressure

Bent hairs

Macula at rest

Sensory hairs

Gelatinous membrane

Displaced macula

Displaced membrane

Pressure

Bent hairs

Examining the ear

The doctor or nurse will use an otoscope to look into your child's ears. This provides a bright light and magnification.

Otoscope

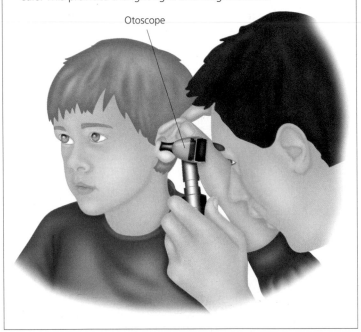

swimmers because dampness in the canal increases the risk of infection. Scratching the inside of the ear with a fingernail or cotton bud can also lead to an external otitis, so it is very important to be extremely gentle when touching a baby's ears. It causes itching and pain in the affected ear and there may also be a discharge from the ear. The infection may be bacterial, viral or fungal.

Treatment for otitis externa

Depending on what is causing the infection, different types of eardrops are prescribed. If the infection is bacterial the drops will contain an antibiotic, but if it is of fungal origin it will contain an antifungal.

Paracetamol may be given to relieve pain and, if it is a viral otitis externa, this may be the only treatment required. The inflammation usually settles down in a few days.

Acute otitis media

This is an inflammation of the middle ear in which there is a collection of fluid, called an effusion, within the middle-ear space. It is a very common problem and each year in the UK about ten per cent of babies aged under three months have an episode of acute otitis media. By the age of three years about thirty per cent of children have been taken to their doctor with acute otitis media.

Otitis media is usually caused by a virus or bacterial infection that has spread via the eustachian tube from the nose or throat after a common cold or sore throat.

Acute otitis media is most common in boys and in children with a family history of ear infections. Certain other groups of children also have frequent infections, including those who live in houses where people smoke, those who have dummies or who are bottle fed (although the reason for this is unclear), and those who have either a history of enlarged adenoids or tonsillitis, or asthma.

This condition causes pain in the ear because the tissues lining the middle ear are inflamed. The inflammation is often accompanied by a high temperature. Young children can be generally unwell and they pull at their ears, which appear to hurt when they are touched. They may also have a partial hearing loss and a discharge from their ear.

Treatment for acute otitis media

- Paracetamol (or ibuprofen) can help to lower a child's temperature and ease pain.

- Your doctor may prescribe antibiotics if the infection is thought to be bacterial in origin. Bacterial infections can result in pus forming in the middle ear, which can be seen with an otoscope, but in about 80 per cent of cases the child recovers in about three days without antibiotics. Serious complications are rare in otherwise healthy children.

Eardrum perforation

Occasionally, if the infection does not clear, fluid in the middle ear continues to build up in this confined space; the increase in pressure inside causes the eardrum to burst and then a discharge will be seen coming from the external canal. The eardrum is said to be 'perforated'.

Treatment for perforated eardrum

These holes often heal up themselves, but, if a child's hearing is affected or if he or she gets repeated ear infections, an operation is performed to repair the hole. A general anaesthetic is given and an overnight stay in hospital is required. After the repair a dressing soaked in antiseptic drops is put in the ear canal and stays in place for two to three weeks, allowing the eardrum to heal. Cotton-wool padding is placed over the ear and held in place with a bandage.

Glue ear

Also known as otitis media with effusion, this is a type of otitis media in which there is an effusion or

Perforated eardrum

A tear or hole on the membrane between the outer and middle ear, usually caused by an acute infection in the middle ear.

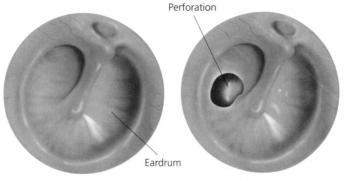

Perforation

Eardrum

Normal eardrum – external view Perforated eardrum

collection of fluid in the middle ear with no signs of infection. It may last for only a short time and cause only a few problems or it may be prolonged. It is common and it has been found that, at any time, five per cent of children aged two to four years have a persistent bilateral (affecting both ears) hearing loss associated with otitis media with effusion.

Children are prone to middle-ear problems because their eustachian tubes are shorter and narrower than in adults. The eustachian tubes become easily blocked if, for example, the adenoids are enlarged or if a child has frequent upper respiratory tract infections. Once the tube is blocked, air can no longer circulate in the middle ear and the fluid becomes thick and sticky, like jelly, and is known as 'glue'.

When this happens the three tiny bones in the middle ear are unable to vibrate freely, dampening down their movement, and a child suffers a mild hearing loss, known as a conductive hearing loss.

Affected children may ask for the television to be turned up or sit very close to it. They may lack concentration and have difficulty with their schoolwork. They can become tired and irritable, their speech may be unclear and they may develop behavioural problems as a result.

Treatment for glue ear

This condition usually clears up itself without treatment. While your child is affected his or her hearing may vary from day to day, so do try to be patient and understanding. If at school, it is also important to discuss the problem with the class teacher so that special arrangements can be made for your child to sit near the teacher, to make sure that he or she can hear everything. However, while present, it is important that a few simple rules are followed:

- Speak clearly to your child but do not shout.

- Look at your child when you are talking to him or her.

- Try to keep background noises down when you are talking to your child.

- If your child's hearing is worse on one side than the other, speak to the child's good side

- Children must be extra careful when crossing a road, because they may not be able to judge traffic distance or direction.

Surgery for glue ear

If a child is being adversely affected by glue ear, he or she may be referred to an ear, nose and throat (ENT) consultant for further assessment. Glue ear is one of the most common reasons for referral for surgery in children in the UK.

If an operation is necessary it is usually carried out under a light, general anaesthetic as a day case. This procedure is known as a myringotomy. The surgeon will make a tiny hole in the eardrum, remove any fluid in the ear and insert a tiny plastic tube, or grommet, into the hole. Grommets remain in the eardrums for about six months to a year. Eventually, the eardrums heal and squeeze the grommet out so that no hole remains in the eardrum.

Children will usually be seen in the outpatient clinic after the operation. If the grommets fall out early or a child continues to have problems, they may need to be re-inserted.

After a grommet operation it is important that a child's ears are kept dry, so earplugs should be used when showering, washing hair or swimming. If a child develops a runny ear the cause may be an infection and this should be checked by the GP.

Air travel

During air travel many adults and children experience some form of ear discomfort. When exposed to changes in pressure the eustachian tube is responsible for equalising the pressure in the middle ear with that of the surrounding environment. In pressurised aircraft cabins this is particularly necessary during take-off and landing. This problem is intensified if there is any upper respiratory tract infection because the opening of the eustachian tube is often narrowed. To try to help relieve the discomfort, it is possible to equalise the middle-ear pressure by yawning, swallowing or chewing.

Glue ear

Normally the middle ear is air filled. If the eustachian tube fails to function normally, the middle ear becomes clogged with mucus. If the condition persists the condition is called 'glue ear'.

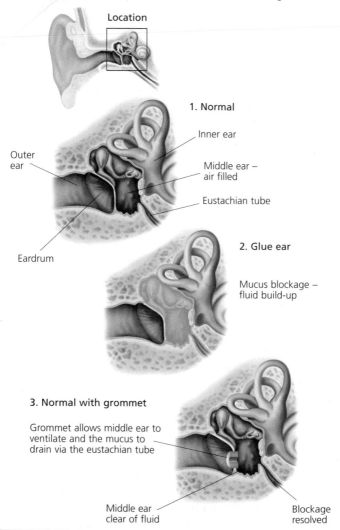

Location

1. Normal

Inner ear

Outer ear

Middle ear – air filled

Eustachian tube

Eardrum

2. Glue ear

Mucus blockage – fluid build-up

3. Normal with grommet

Grommet allows middle ear to ventilate and the mucus to drain via the eustachian tube

Middle ear clear of fluid

Blockage resolved

There is no evidence that giving decongestants to children is helpful, although there is limited evidence that they may be useful in adults.

Hearing problems
The hearing clinic

If a child's hearing is causing concern, he or she will be referred to a hearing clinic (audiology clinic) for tests. There are different ways of testing a child's hearing, depending on the child's age. Once the hearing test has been completed and the doctor has taken all the details about the child's difficulties, his or her ears will be examined using an otoscope, as described earlier.

Testing children aged over four

These children are tested using an instrument called an audiometer. The child wears earphones and listens to a range of precise sounds that are presented through the instrument. Each time the child hears the sound he or she taps on the table to indicate that he or she has heard it. A record of the child's responses is produced and this is known as an audiogram.

The audiogram helps the doctor or audiologist assess whether or not the child's hearing is less good than normal. In addition if there is a loss it will show how severe it is. The test can also indicate whether the loss is the result of a physical problem such as glue ear or of a problem with the nerve that carries impulses from the ear to the brain.

A voice test may also be carried out in which the doctor stands at a specified distance from the child and uses a low voice to say a number of individual words, which the child has to repeat. A score is given for how many of the words are repeated correctly.

Testing children aged under four

Younger children are more difficult to test reliably.
Three year olds are usually tested using the McCormick
toy test: a display of toys is made and the child is asked
to name them. The toys include: a key and tree, a cup
and duck, a person and lamb, a house and cow, a horse
and fork, a plate and plane, and a shoe and spoon.

The child is asked to point to the various toys when
asked, first in a normal conversational voice and then
with the voice at a low level. The child passes the test
if he or she can consistently discriminate between the
items at the low level.

Children younger than three are asked to do a
simple speech test in which they sit on a low chair next
to their carer and when given a small block are asked,
for example, to 'Put it on the table', 'Give it to
Mummy'. The tester stands one metre (three feet)
away at the level of the child's ear. A performance test
may also be carried out where the child has to place a
peg in a board every time he hears a specific sound.

Tympanometry

The final test involves using an instrument called a
tympanometer. This provides information on the
functioning of the middle ear. This is not a painful
procedure and lasts only a minute or two. A probe is
placed in the child's ear canal, which produces sounds
that bounce off the eardrum and are picked up by a
microphone. At the same time pressures in the ear are
varied and the pattern of the reflected waves is recorded
and a graph, or tracing, called a tympanogram is
produced. This is a graph that indicates whether the
eardrum is moving normally and consequently shows if
fluid is present in the middle ear.

Tympanometry

Tympanometry measures the sound-conducting properties of the middle ear. The pressure in the ear canal is raised and lowered while sound waves are projected into the ear. The sound reflected from the eardrum is measured and plotted on a graph.

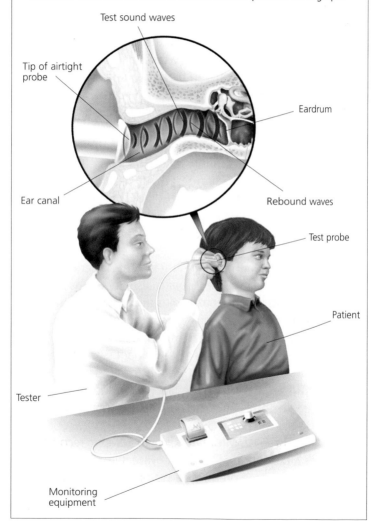

Test sound waves

Tip of airtight probe

Eardrum

Ear canal

Rebound waves

Test probe

Patient

Tester

Monitoring equipment

Newborn baby hearing screening

A small number of babies are born with a hearing loss and it is very important to pick these up as early as possible. In 2005 a new and simple hearing screening test was introduced into most areas of the country and it should be available nationwide in the near future.

The test is carried out within the first few weeks of birth. It does not hurt and only takes a few minutes. In some areas this is offered before your newborn baby leaves the hospital.

A trained hearing technician will place a small earpiece into the baby's ear that sends a clicking sound into the ear. Using a computer, the screener can see how the baby's ear responds to sound. This is known as an otoacoustic emission test (OAE). If a baby has a strong response then he or she is most unlikely to have a hearing loss.

The nose and throat

The upper part of the respiratory system is made up of the nose and throat. The throat is also known as the pharynx and is a tube that begins at the back of the nose (nasopharynx), extends into the back of the mouth (oropharynx), and finally passes to the larynx (laryngopharynx) and into the oesophagus (the tube that carries food and drink through the chest to the stomach). The nose forms the first part of the respiratory system and extends from the nostrils to the nasopharynx.

The tonsils and adenoids

The tonsils are found at the back of the throat (pharynx). Everyone has three areas of tonsillar tissue. The visible tonsils are located on both sides of the back of the throat and look like strawberries; another pair is at the

Otoacoustic testing

Distraction tests cannot be used with a newborn baby. Otoacoustic emission testing detects the presence of 'cochlear echoes', which indicate that the middle and inner ears are healthy. The test is well suited for an infant as it is quick, simple and non-invasive.

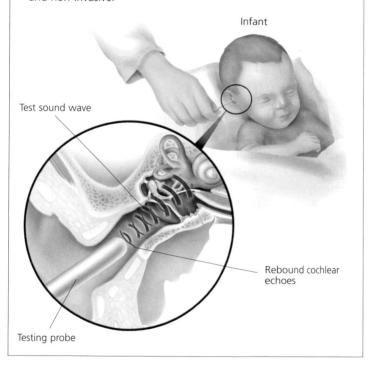

Infant

Test sound wave

Rebound cochlear echoes

Testing probe

base of the tongue and the third pair (commonly referred to as the adenoids) is high up behind the nose.

Tonsils and adenoids are made up of lymphoid tissue, which forms part of the body's immune system. This system helps the body fight infection by producing white blood cells. Tonsils vary in size but are much larger in children than in adults. They are oval in shape and have a pitted surface.

The main tonsils can be easily seen at the back of the throat when the tongue is pressed down by a flat piece of wood, but your doctor can see the adenoids only if he or she looks through a mirror placed at the back of the mouth, or uses a special viewing tube.

Tonsillitis

This is an infection of the tonsils that are visible at the back of the throat and is common in childhood. Some children have repeated episodes of tonsillitis. Viruses or bacteria may cause the infection but the most common cause is a type of bacterium known as *Streptococcus*.

Children with tonsillitis are generally unwell with a high temperature and have difficulty in swallowing. They have enlarged tender glands in their neck. Some children complain of headaches or abdominal pain and may have vomiting or diarrhoea. When a child has tonsillitis the tonsils are reddened and swollen. They may have small white patches on their surface, which is usually indicative of a bacterial infection.

Occasionally a peritonsillar abscess develops, which is known as a quinsy. The symptoms of tonsillitis are severe and swallowing is very painful. The tonsil appears to be displaced towards the midline.

Treatment for tonsillitis

Paracetamol (or ibuprofen) can be used to reduce the fever and ease the pain. Give your child plenty of fluids. If your child does not want to drink, he or she may be tempted to suck an ice-lolly or ice-pop. If a bacterial infection is suspected your doctor will prescribe antibiotics. Most children improve over a few days. As children get older they tend to have fewer episodes of tonsillitis.

Structures of the nose and throat

View into an open mouth

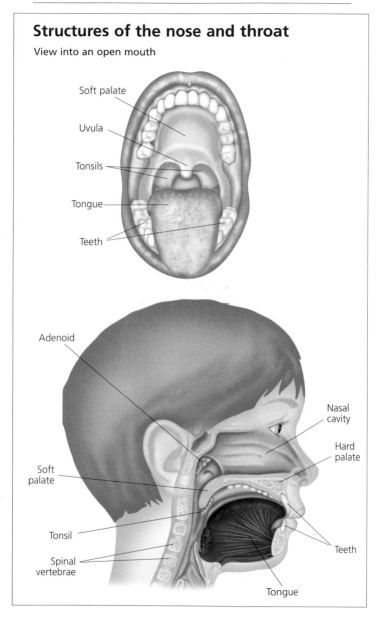

Soft palate

Uvula

Tonsils

Tongue

Teeth

Adenoid

Nasal cavity

Hard palate

Soft palate

Tonsil

Spinal vertebrae

Teeth

Tongue

It is important to note that young children should not gargle because this can spread infection into the middle ear via the eustachian tube.

Surgery for tonsillitis

If a child has more than five episodes of tonsillitis a year they may be referred to an ENT consultant specialist. Removal of the tonsils (tonsillectomy) is likely to be recommended if your child is regularly missing school because of tonsillitis, antibiotics no longer work very well or the enlarged tonsils are interfering with breathing.

The operation is performed under general anaesthetic and a child will usually be allowed home the day after the operation. After the child's tonsils are removed he or she will have a sore throat and the jaw may be stiff; some children complain of earache.

After the operation

- It is very important that children eat and drink as normally as possible and chew solid food. This is difficult at first but soon improves; eating solid food helps to keep the area clean and it will heal more quickly. If children do not eat they are at risk of bleeding and infection.

- Regular pain relief is important and paracetamol or an equivalent should be given.

- Keep your child away from anyone who has an obvious infection for at least a week after the operation. Your child should be kept off school for a minimum of 10 days.

Tonsillectomy

Surgical removal of the tonsils is performed on children who have recurrent episodes of tonsillitis. The operation is performed under general anaesthetic and a child will usually be allowed home the day after the operation.

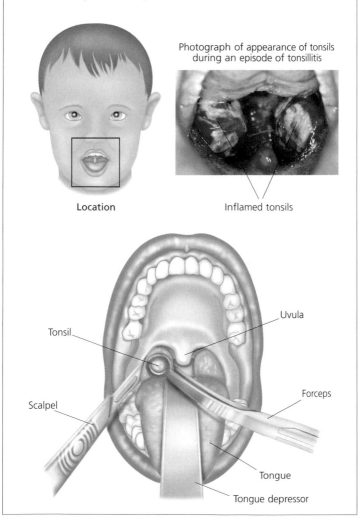

Location

Photograph of appearance of tonsils during an episode of tonsillitis

Inflamed tonsils

Tonsil

Uvula

Scalpel

Forceps

Tongue

Tongue depressor

Enlarged adenoids

Children with large adenoids tend to breathe through their mouths and snore. Enlarged adenoids may cause difficulty with breathing and speech. Affected children may have a very nasal voice and sound as though they have a persistently blocked nose.

If the adenoids partially block the eustachian tube, recurrent middle-ear infections may be a problem. As adenoids shrink naturally with age and almost all are gone by puberty, usually no treatment is required. However, if symptoms are severe, surgical removal may be indicated and an overnight stay in hospital may be required.

Treatment for enlarged adenoids

The adenoids are removed with purpose-built instruments via the mouth and back of the tongue. There are no cuts to the skin. They are often removed at the same time as the tonsils.

Nosebleeds

Very common in children, nosebleeds are often recurrent but usually stop themselves and often occur for no specific reason. They can occur if the lining of the nose is damaged by an injury, perhaps caused by nose picking or forceful nose blowing. Nosebleeds occur if the lining becomes dry and localised areas of inflammation can also lead to bleeding.

Treatment for a nosebleed

Sit your child down and tell him or her to pinch the soft part of the nose for about 10 minutes. Tell the child to spit out any blood in his or her mouth.

Removal of adenoids

The adenoids consist of two areas of lymphatic tissue that form part of the body's defences against infection. If they become enlarged they may cause difficulties with breathing and speech.

1. Before operation

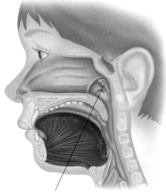

Enlarged adenoid tissue may cause difficulties, for instance with breathing

2. After operation

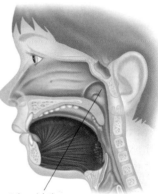

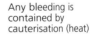

Adenoid tissue removed

Special surgical tools are used through the mouth

Adenoid tissue is cut away

Any bleeding is contained by cauterisation (heat)

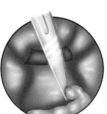

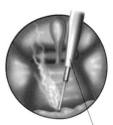

Scalpel (sharp blade)

Adenoids

Cauterising tool

Check the nose and repeat for another 10 minutes. If it is still bleeding after 20 minutes, call for medical advice. Many children appear to grow out of this problem in adolescence. If medical treatment is required, antiseptic cream applied to the nose lining at regular interval appears to be helpful.

If nosebleeds are severe and persistent, cauterisation may be carried out. In this procedure blood vessels are sealed using heat treatment under local anaesthetic. This can be a painful procedure and the results are not always beneficial.

KEY POINTS

■ Ear infections are very common in young children; 80 per cent of cases recover within three days without antibiotics

■ Glue ear is a condition in which there is a collection of fluid in the middle ear, which can result in a fluctuating hearing loss

■ Glue ear often resolves without treatment but in some cases grommets need to be inserted

■ Tonsillitis is usually caused by a bacterial infection

■ Children who have more than five episodes of tonsillitis in one year may be referred to an ear, nose and throat (ENT) specialist

The respiratory tract

Coughs and wheezing in children

Infections of the respiratory tract are extremely common in children. A cough is the most frequent symptom of respiratory disease and many parents seek advice from their doctor because of it.

Listening to a child coughing, particularly during the night, can be very distressing for parents, but in fact coughing serves a useful purpose. Coughing is the body's natural defence mechanism to eliminate phlegm on the chest or mucus from the nose that is trickling down the back of the throat, and is not usually anything to worry about.

As long as your child is still well, feeding, eating and breathing normally, it is usually unnecessary to call a doctor. Wheezing is another common symptom of respiratory disease and is discussed later in the chapter. To understand a little about how these symptoms arise it is useful to know something about the structure of the respiratory system.

The anatomy of the respiratory system

This system extends from the nose, or nasal passages, into the pharynx (throat), larynx (voice box) and main airway, which is known as the trachea or windpipe. The trachea lies at the front of the neck; it is made up of rings of cartilage and has a lining of special cells, which form mucus. This mucus moistens inhaled air and also traps unwanted foreign particles in the airway.

At its base the trachea branches into two tubes known as bronchi. One passes into the right lung and the other into the left. The right bronchus is shorter, wider and more vertical than the left. Each one continues to divide into smaller and smaller tubes called bronchioles, which are like the branches of a tree. Each tiny bronchiole ends in a small balloon-like sac known as an alveolus. These alveoli provide a massive surface area where the gases oxygen and carbon dioxide are exchanged. Each lung contains millions of alveoli.

The lungs themselves are cone shaped, spongy and elastic in texture. Each lung has an apex in the root of the neck and a base that rests on a muscular sheet of tissue, which separates the thorax from the abdomen, called the diaphragm. The lungs are separated from the chest wall by a thin lining known as the pleural membrane, which covers the outside of the ribs and the inside of the chest (thorax). This lining produces a fluid that lubricates these surfaces so that they can slide freely over one another during breathing. The lungs are protected from damage by the ribcage.

Breathing

This is an automatic process controlled by a part of the

The respiratory system

The airways (trachea, bronchi and bronchioles) and airspaces within the lungs supply oxygen to and remove carbon dioxide from the body.

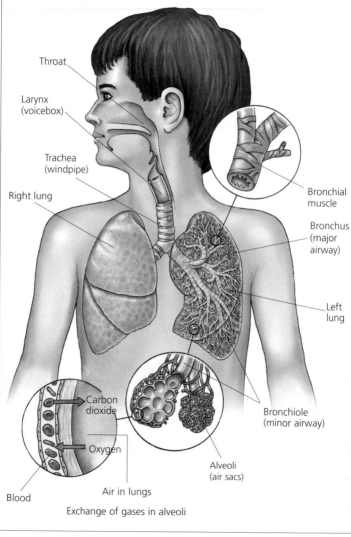

Throat

Larynx (voicebox)

Trachea (windpipe)

Right lung

Bronchial muscle

Bronchus (major airway)

Left lung

Carbon dioxide

Oxygen

Bronchiole (minor airway)

Alveoli (air sacs)

Blood

Air in lungs

Exchange of gases in alveoli

brain known as the respiratory centre. In healthy people it is not something that we are usually aware of.

The respiratory centre stimulates the intercostal muscles, which lie between the ribs, to contract and relax so that the ribcage can move in and out. This process allows air to flow in and out of the lungs.

When you breathe in, the diaphragm and intercostal muscles contract so that the ribcage expands and the diaphragm moves down; each lung expands, taking air containing oxygen into the lungs. When you breathe out the diaphragm and intercostal muscles relax, the ribcage contracts, the diaphragm moves up and each lung decreases in size. This pushes carbon dioxide and unused oxygen out of the lungs.

In this way, tissues in the body receive an adequate supply of oxygen and the waste product of respiration, carbon dioxide, is expelled.

Coughs

There are two types of cough:

1 A dry, irritating cough that causes an itchy feeling at the back of the throat but does not produce phlegm (mucus).

2 A productive or chesty cough that produces phlegm.

Most coughs are the result of viral infections, such as the common cold or influenza, which cause irritation and increased mucus production. Bacterial infections, asthma and exposure to cigarette smoke also cause coughing. An explosive type of cough can be caused by inhalation of a foreign body such as a peanut.

The mechanics of breathing

To inhale air, muscles in the chest wall contract, lifting the ribs and pulling them outwards. The diaphragm moves downward enlarging the chest cavity further. Reduced air pressure in the lungs causes air to enter the lungs from outside. Breathing out reverses this.

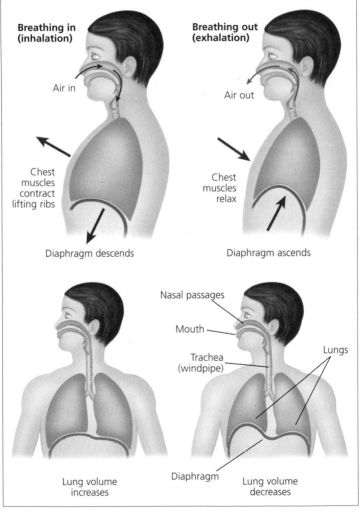

Breathing in (inhalation)

Air in

Chest muscles contract lifting ribs

Diaphragm descends

Breathing out (exhalation)

Air out

Chest muscles relax

Diaphragm ascends

Nasal passages

Mouth

Trachea (windpipe)

Lungs

Diaphragm

Lung volume increases

Lung volume decreases

54

Treatment for coughs

There are many different cough medicines on the market but no scientific study has shown them to be any more effective than a placebo (dummy treatment). A warm drink containing honey and lemon may be helpful for children aged over one year. Giving a child plenty to drink is the most important thing to do and it is essential to avoid smoky atmospheres. Dry atmospheres can aggravate a cough so it may be helpful to place a bowl of water beside a radiator.

Call your doctor if your child has any difficulty breathing or a high temperature, or is producing coloured phlegm because he or she may need antibiotics.

Croup

This is an infection of the upper respiratory tract and is usually caused by a virus. Croup is common in children, particularly between the ages of three months and eight years, and is most frequent during the winter months.

A child with croup has a characteristic dry, barking cough, a hoarse voice and noisy breathing, especially on breathing in (inspiration). This noisy breathing, known as stridor, results from air trying to pass through the narrowed airways. The narrowing is caused by inflammation of the upper airway. A child with croup may also have a mild fever and a runny nose.

Children can have varying degrees of croup, ranging from mild to severe. The symptoms of moderate-to-severe croup can be extremely distressing for a child and the parents.

Treatment for croup

The vast majority of children with croup are treated at home; only about two per cent are admitted to hospital. At home it is felt that breathing in moist air is helpful, although there is no scientific evidence to support this:

- Providing moist air at home is easy enough: take your child into the bathroom, and close the door. Running the hot taps into the bath results in a steamy atmosphere. Sitting your child on your knee and talking to him or her calmly can have a positive effect on the breathing. When the breathing improves take your child back to his or her own room; it may be helpful to increase the humidity in the bedroom by placing a bowl of water near the radiator.

- Children need to be kept well hydrated during an episode of croup, so they should be given plenty to drink.

- If your child has a high temperature give the recommended dose of paracetamol.

Most children recover completely from croup within a few days. Until the age of about eight years croup may recur in a small number of children.

When to seek medical help

If a child does not improve after the steam treatment in the bathroom, medical help should be sought. Signs that suggest the need for medical help are a child having difficulty breathing, with lips or fingernails that appear to be a bluish colour, or a child refusing to drink.

If a child is admitted to hospital, he or she will be given some form of steroids to decrease the inflammation in the airway. A small minority of children may need to be intubated (connected to a ventilator, so that breathing is done for them).

Bronchiolitis

This is the most common lower respiratory tract infection in childhood. In the vast majority of cases bronchiolitis is caused by the respiratory syncytial virus. It is most common during the winter months and generally affects children under one year of age. Parainfluenza virus type 3 is often responsible for bronchiolitis in early spring.

Bronchiolitis causes inflammation in the small tubes in the lungs, the bronchioles. Consequently, the symptoms that children experience are those of airway obstruction. They often have a fever, runny nose, cough, rapid breathing and wheezing that is most obvious when the child breathes out. Children with bronchiolitis tend to sleep for long periods of time because the effort required for the increased number of breaths that they need to take makes them very tired.

Treatment for bronchiolitis

The illness can be mild, moderate or severe. There is no real treatment to kill the virus.

Mild bronchiolitis

When bronchiolitis is mild it can usually be treated at home. Give your child the recommended dose of paracetamol to lower the temperature, and plenty to drink to prevent him or her becoming dehydrated. It is very important that no one smokes in the home, because smoke will make a child's cough and breathing worse. Mild bronchiolitis usually improves and clears up within 10 days.

Severe bronchiolitis

Your child will need to be admitted to hospital. While in hospital your child will be observed closely and made as comfortable as possible. He or she may be given oxygen or inhaled bronchodilator medicine, which helps open the airways.

Nasal secretions will be taken from the child's nose and sent to the laboratory to be tested for viruses and bacteria, to help with the diagnosis. If a child is unable to drink, it may be necessary to give him or her fluids through a small plastic tube that is inserted in a vein until he or she is well enough to drink again.

These more severe cases can last up to three weeks, although there are usually no long-term effects. Premature babies, young babies less than six weeks old and children with congenital heart disease or lung disease are most at risk from developing very severe disease. These children may require admission into an intensive care unit for mechanical ventilation. There is a small percentage of children who may suffer recurrent wheezing for up to five years after bronchiolitis.

Whooping cough

Also known as pertussis, this is a very infectious bacterial infection caused by the bacterium *Bordetella pertussis*. It causes inflammation in the trachea and bronchi and it can be dangerous in children under two years of age.

Before the introduction of the pertussis vaccine, whooping cough caused a considerable number of childhood deaths in the UK. The incidence of this disease has been reduced dramatically by routine immunisation and it is extremely important that children continue to have their immunisations so that the whole population is protected against this disease. Pertussis is now part of the DTaP/IPV/Hib vaccine (introduced in 2006), which is given in three separate doses at two, three and four months of age with a booster dose given between three years and four months and five years (see pages 164–5).

Recognising whooping cough

Whooping cough begins with a runny nose, a mild fever and a persistent cough. After about 10 days the symptoms worsen and the child begins to have severe spasms of coughing, which often end in the characteristic 'whooping' sound on breathing in.

A child may cough up mucus and often vomit after a spasm of coughing. Sometimes young babies do not have the characteristic cough but can appear to be gasping for air, and they can actually stop breathing for a few seconds.

Between coughing spasms the child may seem fine. However, he or she can be very tired, and show loss of appetite and a disturbed sleeping pattern. Some children develop a rash on the face, particularly around the eyes, which results from small blood vessels bursting during a coughing bout.

This phase may last up to six weeks and it may take several weeks to make a full recovery.

Treatment for whooping cough

For most cases there is no treatment that will alter the course of the illness and they recover completely over time.

In severe cases children will need to be admitted to hospital so that oxygen can be given and dehydration prevented. Antibiotics can be given for secondary infections.

Asthma

This is a very common condition that affects about one in seven children in the UK. Children with asthma have airways that are extra sensitive to certain substances, known as triggers, that irritate the airways, causing them to narrow.

Most of the time the child's airways are wide open but, when he or she comes into contact with a trigger, the muscle around the wall of the airway tightens and the internal inflammation causes swelling and mucus production, which narrows the airways. As the airway becomes narrower it becomes more difficult for air to move in and out. Consequently, children who have asthma find breathing difficult.

Recognising asthma

There are four main symptoms of asthma:

1 coughing
2 wheezing
3 chest tightness
4 shortness of breath.

Coughing is typically worse at night or in the early morning. The exact cause of asthma is unknown but a tendency to develop allergies runs in families. Asthma, eczema and hay fever are all allergy-type illnesses and are closely linked.

Asthma triggers

Common triggers for asthma are: house-dust mites, cigarette smoke, viral infections, animals with fur or feathers, pollen, mould spores, paint fumes, exercise,

How asthma affects the airways

During an asthma attack, the muscle walls of the airways contract, causing their internal diameter to narrow. Increased mucus secretion and inflammation of the inner linings of the airways cause further narrowing.

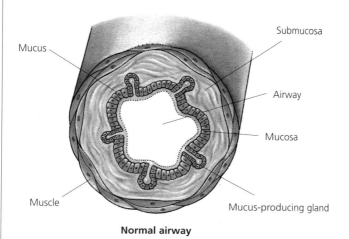

Mucus

Submucosa

Airway

Mucosa

Muscle

Mucus-producing gland

Normal airway

Airway narrows

Swollen submucosa

Muscle contracts

Secretion of mucus from gland increases

Excess mucus

Airway during asthma attack

air temperature, certain foods, laughing, tickling and drugs.

House-dust mites
These are tiny creatures that can be seen only under a microscope. They live in the dust that builds up around the home, so they are found in carpets, beds, soft toys and soft furnishings.

What you can do
It is almost impossible to get rid of all of the house-dust mites in a home but some simple measures can help decrease their numbers:

- Synthetic pillows and duvets should be used.
- Barrier covers should be used for mattresses and pillows.
- Wash bedding weekly at 60°C; this is the temperature required to kill the house-dust mites.
- If you have bunk beds, children with asthma should sleep in the top bunk. Children sleeping in a bottom bunk are exposed to many more house-dust mite allergens as they continually fall from the mattress above.
- Put soft toys in the freezer for 24 hours every 2 weeks to kill the mites and again wash at 60°C to remove dead mites.
- Carpets should be vacuumed frequently.
- Clean surfaces with a damp cloth at least once a week.
- Humidity levels should be kept to a minimum by keeping rooms well aired.

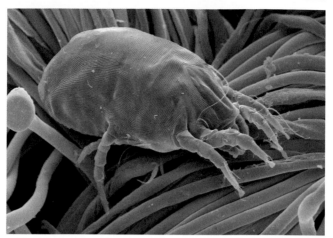

The house-dust mite, shown here on the woven threads of a textile, is smaller than a full stop on this page. Dust mites live in carpets, mattresses and other soft furnishings. Their dead bodies and faeces can trigger asthma.

If these simple measures seem to be ineffective, other more expensive measures can be tried, for example, replacing carpets with laminate flooring and curtains with blinds.

Cigarette smoke
This is a major trigger of asthma symptoms, so, if a child has asthma, he or she must not be exposed to it.

What you can do
If either parent smokes it must be a priority to stop. If this is not possible, the parent should not smoke in the house or anywhere around the child.

Viral infections
Colds and other viral infections are common triggers in young children but are very difficult to avoid.

What you can do
Using the correct asthma medication as prescribed can reduce the risk of an asthma attack. Increasing medication at the first sign of an infection can stop deterioration. Once the infection has cleared the usual dose of medication can be taken.

Pets
Allergy to cats and dogs triggers asthma symptoms in 50 per cent of children with asthma. Although any furry animal can trigger asthma, occasionally birds also cause symptoms.

What you can do
It is obviously best not to keep pets at all but, if a family already has one, the next best thing to do is to keep animals out of the bedrooms and bath them thoroughly once a week. In severe cases, the animal may have to be adopted by someone else.

Pollen
There are many different types of pollen grains from trees, grasses and plants, and individual children can be sensitive to different ones. It can be very difficult to avoid pollen, particularly in the spring and summer months.

What you can do
It is important to avoid spending too much time outside on hot sunny days if your child is sensitive to grass pollen. Children who are sensitive to grass pollen should not play in long grass, and should stay inside, with the windows closed, when the grass is being cut.

Mould spores

Mould grows in any warm, damp place. It is common in damp houses, particularly in bathrooms and kitchens. Moulds release tiny seeds called spores into the air; it is these that can trigger asthma symptoms.

What you can do

To reduce humidity in the home, keep rooms well ventilated and windows should be opened after cooking or a bath or shower, and wet clothes should not be dried inside the home. If mould does appear, remove it as quickly as possible with a special mould-removing cleaner.

Exercise

Some children find that exercise triggers their symptoms. However, exercise is good for everyone and children with asthma should be able to exercise without difficulty.

What you can do

If a child takes his or her asthma medication properly, exercise will be possible. A child should take two puffs of the reliever inhaler 10 to 15 minutes before exercise and this should help prevent any symptoms developing. Extra care needs to be taken on cold, dry days and especially if a child has a cold or other infection. Swimming is a very good form of exercise for anyone with asthma because the air in the pool is warm and moist and, when exposed for a short period of time, helps to decrease airway sensitivity.

Air temperature

Sudden changes in temperature, cold air and wind can all affect children with asthma.

What you can do
Remind your child to take a dose of reliever before going out into the cold, and wrap a scarf around the child's face. If a bedroom is too warm and a child is over-wrapped, this can also worsen asthma symptoms.

Foods
Food allergy is uncommon but certain foods can exacerbate asthma symptoms. Dairy products, shellfish, fish, yeast products and nuts are some of the offenders.

What you can do
Avoid those foods that appear to make a child's asthma symptoms worse.

Drugs
In a few cases some medicines can lead to an asthma attack. Aspirin and ibuprofen are two examples.

What you can do
Give paracetamol to a child with a fever (not ibuprofen). No child under the age of 16 should be given aspirin anyway because of a small risk of it causing a rare but very serious disease, Reye's syndrome.

Long-term treatment for asthma
The main goal of asthma treatment is for a child to be symptom free day and night. Children with asthma should be able to lead completely normal lives and with the correct treatment this should be possible.

Most asthma medication is given via an inhaler so that the medicine is breathed in and goes straight to the lungs where it is required. There are two main types of inhalers: relievers and preventers. Reliever inhalers are used to help breathing difficulties when they occur, whereas preventer inhalers help protect the airways and reduce the possibility of developing asthma symptoms.

Young children do not have the coordination necessary to use an inhaler properly and therefore spacer devices are used. These are large plastic containers that are put on to the inhaler before use. The medicine is trapped inside the spacer and allows the child to breathe it in at his or her own pace.

The spacer must be kept clean and should be washed with soapy water and allowed to drip-dry after use.

Reliever inhalers

Every child with asthma should have a reliever inhaler. When taken as soon as asthma symptoms appear, the medicine quickly relaxes the muscles surrounding the narrowed airways. This allows the airways to open wider, making it easier for air to move in and out of the lungs. If taken before exercise inhalers can also decrease the chances of a child becoming wheezy.

Reliever inhalers are usually blue and the most common are salbutamol (Ventolin) and terbutaline (Bricanyl). They usually have an effect in five to ten minutes. If an attack is particularly bad, the reliever may have to be given again, but if this is the case medical advice should be obtained as soon as possible. Some children require a longer-lasting reliever, the main one being salmeterol (Serevent). This tends to be given on a regular basis along with a preventer.

Preventer inhalers

Medication in these inhalers protects the lining of the

Spacer devices

Allow the patient to concentrate on breathing in the medication rather than having to coordinate inhaling and pressing the inhaler button at the same time.

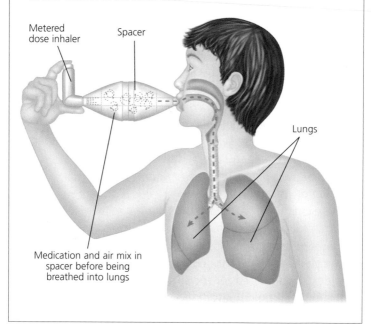

Metered dose inhaler

Spacer

Lungs

Medication and air mix in spacer before being breathed into lungs

airways. They decrease the sensitivity of the lining so that when the airway comes into contact with a trigger it reacts less dramatically, with the result that the swelling and inflammation are decreased.

Preventer inhalers are usually brown or orange and the most common are budesonide (Pulmicort), beclometasone (Becotide) and fluticasone (Flixotide). They are all inhaled steroids and take about 14 days to become effective. They will usually be prescribed if a child needs to use a reliever more than once a day on a regular basis.

Sodium cromoglicate (Intal) is also an inhaled preventer but not a steroid. It needs to be taken several times a day and is not usually as effective as inhaled steroids.

Regular use of preventers is important

Preventer medication reduces the risk of a severe attack but does not bring immediate relief from symptoms. The protective effect builds up over time so that it is important that children take them every day, usually every morning and evening. Parents sometimes forget to give the preventer regularly. To help remember it is best to give it at the same time each day, for example, make it a part of a regular routine such as before cleaning teeth in the morning and evening.

Steroids for asthma

Many parents worry about giving their child steroids. It is important to know that the steroids used to treat asthma are corticosteroids, which are copies of those produced naturally in the body. They are very different to the anabolic steroids that are sometimes used by body builders and athletes. Inhaled steroids pass directly into the lungs so that little is absorbed into the rest of the body. Low doses of inhaled steroids do not affect growth and should not cause side effects.

A short course of steroid tablets, usually prednisolone, may be needed to treat a particularly severe attack. They are given for only about five days so that side effects are not usually experienced.

Peak-flow meters

These are used to measure a child's lung performance

by measuring how fast air can be blown out of the lungs. This in turn indicates how wide the airways are at the time of the test and can therefore help to identify warning signs of worsening asthma. Peak-flow readings tend to fall when asthma is worsening. It is best to record peak-flow readings twice each day, once in the morning and once in the evening. It is not necessary to do this all the time but only if directed by the asthma nurse or doctor, when treatment is changed and when an attack is suspected.

Peak-flow meter

A peak-flow meter measures your peak expiratory flow (PEF) – how fast you can blow out after taking a deep breath of air. This gives useful clues about the present state of your asthma.

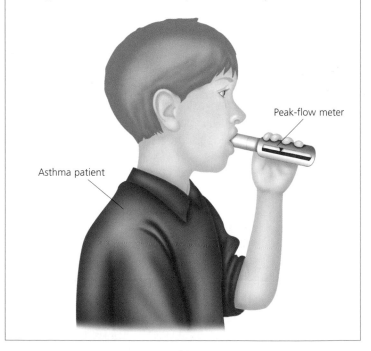

Peak-flow meter

Asthma patient

Nebulisers

These are machines that create a mist of medicine that the child breathes in through a mask or mouthpiece. These are rarely needed at home for asthma now because inhalers and spacers are so effective. Nebulisers are used mainly in hospitals, but in certain circumstances can be used at home and may be recommended by the hospital consultant if, for example, your child has severe asthma or cannot use a spacer.

How nebulisers work

The nebuliser is a simple air compressor. It bubbles air through a solution of the drug, generating a mist, which is inhaled through either a mask or a mouthpiece.

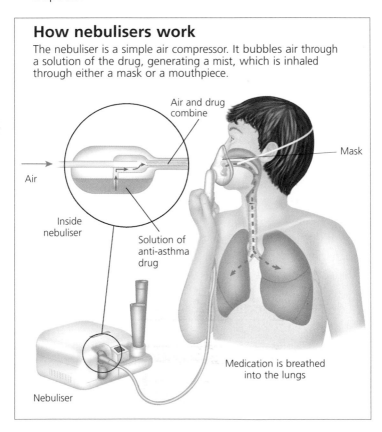

Air and drug combine

Mask

Air

Inside nebuliser

Solution of anti-asthma drug

Medication is breathed into the lungs

Nebuliser

Treating an asthma attack

Asthma symptoms are often mild, but occasionally symptoms are more severe and urgent treatment is required:

- A child should be given his or her reliever and you need to stay calm and reassuring.

- Help your child to sit upright.

- Encourage him or her to breathe slowly and calmly.

- Any tight clothing should be loosened.

The reliever should work within five to ten minutes, but if it does not it should be repeated. The following are danger signs during an attack:

- The child is distressed and unable to talk.
- The child is becoming exhausted.
- The child's lips are going blue.
- The child's breathing does not improve after using the reliever inhaler.

If this is the situation, call your doctor or the emergency services for an ambulance and continue to repeat the reliever while waiting for help to arrive.

Long-term prognosis for asthma

It is difficult to say for certain whether a child will grow out of asthma. Research has shown that about a third of children with asthma find that their symptoms disappear by the time that they are adults. Others will find that their symptoms become milder. Some children find that they get better during adolescence, but their symptoms may return in later life. For a fuller account of asthma see another title in this series, the Family Doctor Book *Understanding Asthma*.

KEY POINTS

■ Most coughs in children are the result of viral infections

■ Croup is an infection of the upper respiratory tract

■ Bronchiolitis is the most common lower respiratory tract infection (in young children) and more serious cases need to be treated in hospital

■ Before the introduction of the pertussis vaccine, whooping cough caused a considerable number of childhood deaths

■ One in seven children is affected by asthma

■ There are many common asthma triggers; most of them can be controlled (to a certain extent)

■ The main goal of asthma treatment is for a child to be symptom free day and night

■ In treatment of asthma, preventer inhalers protect the lining of the airways, whereas relievers quickly relax the muscles surrounding them

The gastrointestinal tract

The scope of gastrointestinal illness

Diarrhoea and vomiting are the most common symptoms of gastrointestinal illness. The rapidity with which diarrhoea and vomiting spread through families, nurseries and schools is always a concern for parents (and teachers). This is particularly so in a large family when parents try their hardest to halt it, but, very often, one child after another gets it, despite the parents' best efforts. Parents often end up with it too!

At the other end of the spectrum are children suffering from constipation, which appears to be an increasing problem.

Abdominal pain or 'tummy ache' is not as common in children as in adults. Young children especially may complain of 'tummy ache' but the pain could be anywhere in the body because they have difficulty in identifying the source of pain.

Colic and gastro-oesophageal reflux are also common problems in babies.

Anatomy of the gastrointestinal tract

The gastrointestinal tract is the main part of the digestive system (the other parts being the organs associated with it, the pancreas, gallbladder and liver). It is a convoluted (much folded) muscular tube, which extends from the mouth to the anus. It is approximately 7 metres (23 feet) long. It comprises:

- The oesophagus (or gullet), which leads from the mouth to the stomach
- The stomach
- The small intestine: divided into three parts – the duodenum, jejunum and ileum
- The large intestine: divided into the colon and rectum.

Each part of the gastrointestinal tract plays its part in digesting food into simple components or nutrients, which the body uses for energy, growth and tissue repair. Any remaining waste is discarded as faeces.

The digestion of food

Digestion begins in the mouth where food is chewed and broken down into small pieces and mixed with saliva. It is then swallowed, when it passes into the oesophagus and on into the stomach. The stomach has valves or sphincters, one at its entrance and one at the exit, that help keep the food inside so that further digestion can occur. The stomach's juices contain acid and chemicals or enzymes. These substances, together with the rhythmic movements of the stomach, convert food and drink into a liquid called chyme.

When digestion in the stomach is complete, the sphincter at the outlet of the stomach relaxes (opens) and allows small amounts of chyme into the

The major abdominal organs and digestion

Ingested food passes down the oesophagus and into the stomach, where it is mixed thoroughly with digestive juices secreted by the stomach lining. Further digestive juices are added to the food in the duodenum.

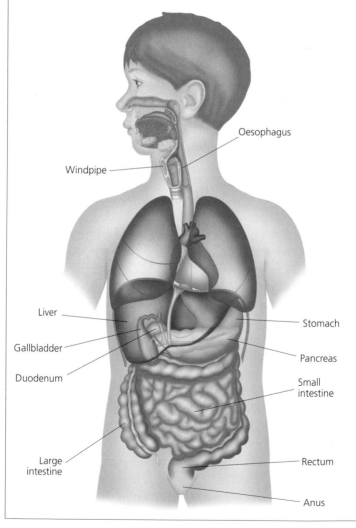

Windpipe

Oesophagus

Liver

Stomach

Gallbladder

Duodenum

Pancreas

Small intestine

Large intestine

Rectum

Anus

duodenum, which is the first part of the small intestine. In here special fluid from the pancreas and bile from the gallbladder are added to the chyme to break it down even further. In the remaining part of the small intestine even more enzymes are added, and the chyme is broken down into nutrients and water that can be absorbed into the bloodstream so that it can be circulated around the body.

The material passing from the small intestine into the large intestine consists of water and undigested matter such as roughage. There are no enzymes in the large intestine and no digestion takes place here. It does, however, absorb water and semi-solid waste, or faeces, is formed. Faeces are expelled at intervals through the anus.

Constipation

Constipation is a very common problem in children and is characterised by difficulty or delay in the passage of stools, which are often, but not always, hard. Everyone has a different bowel pattern so some children may open their bowels once or twice each day, whereas others may open theirs only once every two or three days. Each of these can be considered normal. A bowel pattern becomes a problem only if it is causing other symptoms.

What causes constipation?

Constipation occurs for a variety of reasons. In babies and toddlers it is often because a child is not having enough water to drink. The stools consequently become dried up and hard:

- When a child has a minor illness, such as a cold,

    there is an increased need for the body to retain

The digestive process

Food passes from the stomach into the small intestine, where absorption of nutrients begins. The large intestine comes after the small intestine, and absorbs water and eliminates undigested waste.

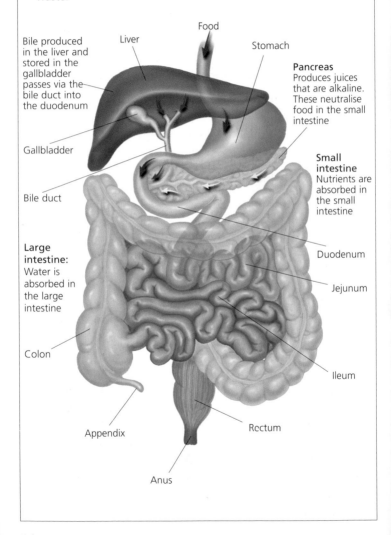

Food

Liver

Stomach

Bile produced in the liver and stored in the gallbladder passes via the bile duct into the duodenum

Pancreas
Produces juices that are alkaline. These neutralise food in the small intestine

Gallbladder

Small intestine
Nutrients are absorbed in the small intestine

Bile duct

Large intestine:
Water is absorbed in the large intestine

Duodenum

Jejunum

Colon

Ileum

Appendix

Rectum

Anus

fluid and so the stools become harder and less frequent.

- Occasionally, an anal fissure, which is a small tear around the anus, occurs after passing a large stool, which can hurt every time that the child opens his or her bowels. This results in a child 'holding' on for longer, which leads to larger, harder stools that cause even more discomfort when they are eventually passed. A vicious circle is set up that can be very difficult to break.

- If your child dislikes the school toilets, he or she may 'hold on' until he or she returns home and this will have a similar outcome.

- A diet low in fibre will also lead to hard stools (faeces) (whereas a diet high in fibre combined with regular water intake helps stools become large and soft).

- Soiling – the involuntary passage of fluid or semi-solid stool into clothing – is usually the result of overflow from an overfull rectum.

Encopresis caused by constipation

'Encopresis' is the term used to describe the passage of stools in inappropriate places (for example, on the floor or into clothing) occurring at least once a month for three months or more in children aged over four years. It is usually the result of constipation and can be described as either a primary problem, where the child has never established bowel control, or a secondary problem, where children have had control for at least six months before its onset. Over half the cases of encopresis are secondary. Encopresis is four or five times more common in boys than in girls and usually resolves spontaneously by adolescence.

Treatment for constipation

This involves general advice and routines around toileting. There are general tips to follow and in some cases medication can be given.

General tips
Food

What children eat affects bowel regularity. Eating large amounts of dairy products, chocolate and biscuits can cause constipation, whereas eating foods high in fibre may improve it. Fibre-rich foods such as brown bread, apples and dried fruit can be helpful but it must be remembered that, if extra fibre is eaten, extra fluid must be drunk.

Children should eat at regular times and eat about the same amount of food at each meal so that the bowel can establish a regular rhythm.

Exercise

Regular exercise promotes regular bowel movements.

Toileting routine

Establish a routine to try to produce a regular bowel habit. Children should be encouraged to sit on the toilet about 15 to 20 minutes after a meal, for about 5 to 10 minutes at most. They should never be made to sit there for longer than this.

It is important that you watch your child's attempts to pass a stool. Some children sit quite passively and do not make any attempt to push down into their bottoms as they need to do. Remain calm and encouraging throughout, because this will be far more effective than becoming angry and impatient.

Medical treatment

If, after having followed the above advice, there has been no improvement, it is advisable to consult your doctor, who may recommend the use of laxatives.

Laxatives

There are different types of laxatives used to treat constipation. Over-the-counter laxatives are not recommended for children. Always seek advice from your doctor or pharmacist.

- Lactulose: this is one of the most common initial treatments and works by softening the stools. It is a simple sugar that is not broken down in the small bowel but digested by bacteria that are naturally present in the large bowel. It draws water into the colon and keeps the stool softer for longer.

- Senna and picolax: these laxatives work in a completely different way. They make the gut muscles contract more powerfully and help push the stool along the bowel. Some abdominal discomfort can occur with these.

- Movicol: this is another different kind of laxative, which works by keeping fluid within the bowel and consequently produces a softer stool.

Enemas and suppositories

Enemas (introduction of a solution into the rectum and colon) and suppositories (a medicine placed in the rectum) have been widely used to treat constipation but it is now thought that such an unpleasant treatment may have an adverse psychological effect on a child. However, your child's doctor may feel that it is essential to use them if a child has an impacted bowel, which requires clearing before a regular bowel pattern can be established.

Biofeedback

This treatment method can be used for children who have poor sensations of rectal filling and are unsure about which sensations to react to. It teaches children how to tell when they need to open their bowels and how to relax the right muscles to let the stool out.

A machine is used to measure how tight the muscles around a child's anus and rectum are. Thin probes are placed inside the anus and rectum and the probes send information to a computer. The child squeezes in his or her anus and then relaxes as if passing a stool. The computer displays the pattern as sounds or pictures. Children then have to practise passing a stool. The probe has a small balloon on it and when filled with air gives the child the urge to pass a stool. The child learns to use the cues from the sounds or pictures on the computer to train the muscles to tighten and relax in the right way.

It can take a long time to learn this biofeedback method and there is not too much evidence that it always works.

Colic

Infantile colic is the term used to describe excessive crying in an otherwise healthy baby. By definition excessive crying is crying that lasts at least three hours a day, for three days a week, for at least three weeks. When the baby cries it seems to have a pain in the tummy and may be accompanied by drawing up of the legs to the abdomen. Colic typically starts in the first few weeks of life and has nearly always cleared up by the time the baby is four to five months old. It often occurs in the evening.

This is a common problem that prompts one in six families to consult a health professional for advice because it causes real distress and anxiety. Although the exact cause of colic remains unknown, we do know that it is not a disease and is not caused by any fault in parental care. A variety of reasons for it have been put forward. It may simply be normal that some babies cry a little, whereas others cry a great deal. Possible explanations include painful contractions of the gut, wind or a transient intolerance to lactose, which is the natural sugar found in milk.

Management of colic

Simple reassurance that a baby is not ill and that the colic will stop within a few months is perhaps the most important message for parents. You need to check that your baby is not hungry, thirsty, unwell or uncomfortable. Do not change from breast to bottle or switch from one formula to another if bottle-feeding. Medicines used for colic are not usually effective.

Increasing the amount of time that you carry your baby does not seem to help. Scientific trials looking at possible helpful treatments have been inconclusive. Either the studies have been too small to reach a definite conclusion or there has been contradictory evidence, some studies suggesting that a particular treatment works whereas another says that it does not.

As yet the effectiveness of the following treatments is unknown: low-lactose milk, sucrose solution, infant massage, cranial osteopathy, spinal manipulation, herbal tea and reducing infant stimulation. Further studies need to be carried out to ascertain what really is effective to reduce the distress and anxiety caused to both babies and parents by colic.

Gastro-oesophageal reflux

This occurs in two forms: simple gastro-oesophageal reflux or posseting and gastro-oesophageal reflux disease.

Simple gastro-oesophageal reflux

In this case small amounts of milk come up into the baby's mouth. This is extremely common, but parents can become anxious about it. If your baby is well, thriving and has no other symptoms, you can be reassured that this will improve in time.

Treatment for simple reflux

Advice for parents with a baby who has simple reflux includes:

- If you are bottle-feeding, check that the teat size is correct for your child's age.
- Make sure that you tilt the bottle correctly so that the baby is not swallowing air as well as milk.
- Ensure that the baby is not having too much milk at one feed.
- Feed the baby in a more upright position.

Gastro-oesophageal reflux disease

This is a condition in which the acid contents of the stomach reflux, or pass up, into the oesophagus or gullet. This happens when the valve at the lower end of the oesophagus relaxes, allowing the gastric contents to flow in the wrong direction out of the stomach. When this happens infants can experience recurrent vomiting, abdominal pain, feeding difficulties or failure to thrive, and they may be generally irritable. These symptoms

Gastro-oesophageal reflux

This symptom occurs when the stomach contents leak out of the stomach into the oesophagus. This happens when the valve at the top of the stomach fails to remain tightly closed.

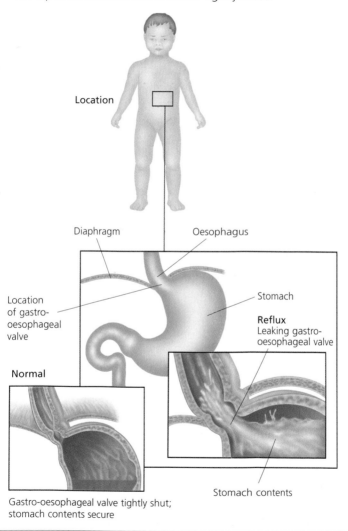

Location

Diaphragm

Oesophagus

Location of gastro-oesophageal valve

Stomach

Reflux
Leaking gastro-oesophageal valve

Normal

Stomach contents

Gastro-oesophageal valve tightly shut; stomach contents secure

occur because the acid from the stomach causes inflammation of the lining of the oesophagus.

Premature babies are particularly prone to develop symptoms as well as babies who have been born with an abnormality of the oesophagus. Babies with a hiatus hernia are also at risk of this problem – this is a condition in which part of the stomach passes into the chest through a weakened part of the diaphragm (the muscle dividing the chest cavity from the abdominal cavity).

Most babies with gastro-oesophageal reflux disease improve spontaneously by 12 to 18 months of age, but, if symptoms are associated with a hiatus hernia, it may persist until the age of four years.

Treatment for gastro-oesophageal reflux disease
Many different treatments are used to help infants with reflux disease, but the true effectiveness of most of these is unknown. Some parents may be tempted to lie their young babies on their sides or to lie them on their front to try to help prevent reflux, but this sleeping position carries an increased risk of sudden infant death syndrome (cot death) and consequently should never be tried.

The situation with gastro-oesophageal reflux disease is similar to that for colic, in which studies are either too small to draw any meaningful conclusion or different studies produce conflicting results. Some of these treatments may work for some babies, as below, whereas others will produce no benefit at all.

Feed thickeners
As their name implies these simply thicken the milk so that it is less likely to regurgitate into the oesophagus.

Hiatus hernia

The hiatus is a small hole in the muscular diaphragm through which the oesophagus passes. If there is a weakness in the hiatus, part of the stomach may slide into the chest – causing a hiatus hernia.

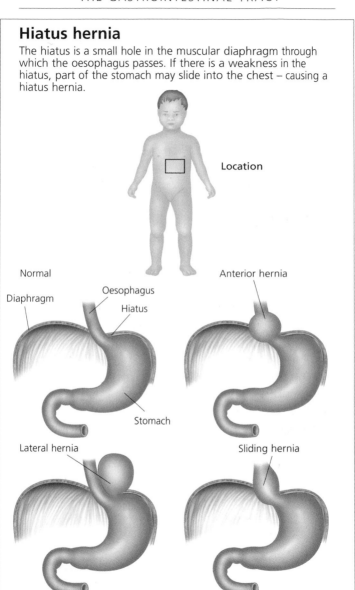

Location

Normal

Diaphragm

Oesophagus

Hiatus

Stomach

Anterior hernia

Lateral hernia

Sliding hernia

Alginates
These form a layer that floats on the top of the stomach contents to decrease reflux into the oesophagus.

Medicines
Cimetidine decreases the amount of acid in the stomach so that less damage is caused to the oesophageal lining when reflux occurs. Metoclopramide and domperidone are medicines used to relieve nausea and vomiting. These medicines all have to be prescribed by your doctor.

Gastroenteritis
Acute gastroenteritis is an inflammation of the lining of the stomach and intestines. It causes a rapid onset of diarrhoea, which is usually accompanied by vomiting. It can also cause abdominal pain, fever and nausea. Diarrhoea does not mean passing the occasional loose stool. It is defined as the frequent passage of unformed liquid stools.

Gastroenteritis is very common and in less developed countries it causes four million deaths per year in children under the age of five years. In the developed world close to 90 per cent of cases are caused by viruses, the most common one being the rotavirus.

This virus can affect all children, but babies and children up to two years of age are most vulnerable. Bacteria cause most of the remaining cases and these are predominantly *Campylobacter, Salmonella* and *Shigella* species, and *Escherichia coli (E. coli)*.

The infection may be acquired from contaminated food or water. Outbreaks commonly occur within families and people who are in close contact as the viruses and bacteria are passed from one person to another.

Preventing gastroenteritis

It is therefore very important to wash hands thoroughly to prevent the spread of gastroenteritis, especially:

- before preparing food
- after using the toilet, or helping your child use the toilet
- after changing your baby's nappy.

It is also important to clean bottles, teats and feeding equipment thoroughly after each feed for babies aged less than one year. Wash everything in hot soapy water using bottle and teat brushes as soon as possible after they have been used, and then they should be rinsed thoroughly and stored in a sterilising solution.

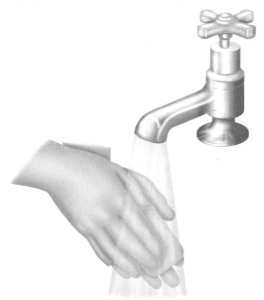

Wash your hands and nails thoroughly to prevent the spread of infection.

Disinfect contaminated surfaces and wash soiled clothes promptly.

Treatment for gastroenteritis

As viruses cause most cases of gastroenteritis antibiotics are unhelpful. Children should not be given medicines to stop diarrhoea because these may exert harmful side effects. For example, they can affect breathing, lower blood pressure and alter the heart rate.

One of the most serious consequences of diarrhoea and vomiting in babies and children is dehydration and the prevention of this is the mainstay of treatment.

Children who have gastroenteritis should be encouraged to swallow frequent small volumes of an oral rehydration fluid, such as Dioralyte, to replace the fluid and mineral salts lost through vomiting or diarrhoea.

Make the solution exactly as directed and keep it in the fridge. It should be discarded after 24 hours. If too little or too much water is used to make up the solution, it will either make the medicine less effective or cause a salt imbalance.

Soft drinks, such as lemonade or cola, alone are inappropriate. If rehydration fluids are unavailable, plain water should be used.

If you are breast-feeding a baby, feeding should be continued and the extra fluid lost replaced with oral rehydration fluids given from a spoon or a liquid medicine measure.

Bottle-fed babies can alternate between their usual formula feeds and rehydration fluids.

For children on a mixed diet offer their usual foods, but it is thought best if they eat and drink less milk products during the attack. Oral rehydration fluids should again be given to replace losses.

If vomiting continues it is best to give very little, very often, for example, one teaspoon every five to ten minutes.

Normal feeding should be resumed as soon as possible because there is no evidence that fasting will have any benefit. Eating foods that are high in carbohydrates, such as bread, pasta or potatoes, is helpful to aid recovery.

When to seek medical help

Although most children recover quickly from gastroenteritis with no long-lasting effects, if you notice any of the following signs of dehydration medical advice should be sought immediately.

- Drowsiness
- Dry lips, mouth and tongue
- Sunken fontanelle (baby's soft spot on the top of the head)
- Sunken eyes
- No tears
- Reduced elasticity of the skin: watching what happens when the skin is pinched can show this; if a child is dehydrated the skin will stay up when pinched
- Reduced urine output: this is identified when a child has persistently dry nappies.

Toddler's diarrhoea

This condition affects children between the ages of one and five years. These children are generally healthy and eat and grow well, but they pass frequent, smelly, loose stools. Their stools characteristically contain undigested food, such as peas and pieces of carrot, which often appear within hours of eating them.

Although the exact cause of toddler's diarrhoea is unknown, dietary factors have been implicated. The diet of infants and toddlers has changed dramatically over recent years and many studies have shown that constant fluid intake, low dietary fat and an excessive consumption of fruit juice have replaced a traditional well-balanced diet and may be contributing to the increased incidence of toddler's diarrhoea.

Treatment for toddler's diarrhoea

If a child is well and growing normally, parents can be reassured that there is no underlying illness and the child will get better in time.

A change in a child's diet often helps improve the situation and the following simple measures are often effective within days:

- Excessive amounts of fruit juices and squash should be avoided; give your child milk or water instead.

- Switching from a bottle to a cup helps reduce the amount of fluid drunk.

- Clear apple juice causes a particular problem and should be replaced with cloudy apple juice.

- Fat intake should be increased, for example, by using whole cream milk, adding butter to foods and avoiding low fat foods.

- Although the excessive use of fibre should be avoided, children should be encouraged to eat a variety of fruit and vegetables.

Threadworms

These are tiny white worms, which are about a centimetre (half an inch) long and look like pieces of cotton. They live in the bowel and around the anus and they are a very common problem, particularly in children. They do not cause any serious damage but they can be irritating. It is estimated that approximately 40 per cent of children aged under 10 may be infected at any one time and many of these have no symptoms.

Threadworms produce large numbers of tiny eggs, which are so small that they cannot be seen with the naked eye. They are present in house dust, carpets, towels and bed linen, and can easily be picked up on the fingers and swallowed. Once this happens, the eggs pass into the bowel where they hatch into worms.

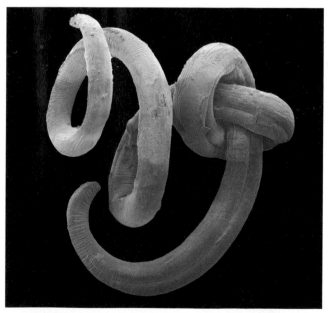

A threadworm photographed under a microscope.

When mature the female worms migrate to the anus and lay eggs there at night; it is this that causes the itchiness. Children scratch themselves and the eggs are transferred on to fingers and under fingernails. Eggs can easily get into the mouth again, for example, by thumb sucking or nail biting, which causes re-infection. They can also spread to other members of the family by direct contact, food and shared use of towels and linens.

Treatment for threadworms

Treatment involves taking a single dose of medicine (obtained on prescription from your doctor), which kills the worms. As threadworms spread so easily, it is essential that all family members be treated at the same time. Underwear, nightwear, towels and bed linen should be washed as soon as everyone has been

Preventing re-infection with threadworms

It is important that you take the following steps to prevent re-infection:

- Keep fingernails short
- Wash hands thoroughly after going to the toilet and before eating
- Discourage nail biting
- Wear pyjamas or underclothes in bed
- Make sure everyone bathes daily
- Change clothes and wash bed linen regularly
- Ensure that each family member uses only his or her own towel

treated. Carpets should be vacuumed and bedrooms dusted or wiped down with a clean damp cloth.

KEY POINTS

■ Constipation is characterised by difficulty or delay in the passage of stools

■ Simple dietary changes should be tried as a first-line treatment for constipation

■ Laxatives should be used only under the supervision of the GP

■ The exact cause of colic is unknown but it is self-limiting and always resolves by six months of age

■ Simple gastro-oesophageal reflux is common and self-limiting

■ Gastro-oesophageal disease is more problematic but a variety of treatments is available

■ It is important to be able to recognise the signs of dehydration so that medical advice can be sought immediately

The urinary system

Anatomy of the urinary system

Urinary tract infections and bedwetting are the most frequent problems associated with the urinary tract.

The urinary tract consists of the kidneys, ureters, bladder and urethra. The kidneys are reddish brown, bean-shaped organs that lie on either side of the spine at the back of the abdomen. In an adult they are about 10 to 12.5 cm (4 to 5 inches) long and 5 to 7.5 cm (2 to 3 inches) wide. Urine formed in the kidneys passes into the bladder via two thin, muscular tubes known as ureters, approximately 25 to 30 cm (10 to 12 inches) long.

Urine is stored in a hollow muscular organ called the bladder located in the pelvis, and excreted at intervals through a tube called the urethra.

The amount that a bladder can hold before it needs emptying varies and is called the 'functional bladder capacity', for example, an adult will have an average capacity of 420 millilitres or ml (15 fluid ounce or fl oz), a 12-year-old child 330 ml (11.5 fl oz) and a 7 year old 240 ml (8.5 fl oz). A frequent need to go to the toilet is a sign of a low functional bladder capacity.

Purpose of the kidneys

The kidneys basically act as filters to 'clean the blood' and they have three main functions:

1 They remove a substance called urea, which is a byproduct of digestion.
2 They regulate the salt content of the blood.
3 They adjust the water content of the body.

For the body to perform properly it is essential that these three functions are maintained at constant levels, and this makes the work of the kidneys extremely important.

Water is taken into the body as food and drink and is lost in two main ways: in urine and sweat. So, for example, on a cold day, when you do not need to sweat, your urine is pale, dilute and there is a lot of it; on a hot day, because you sweat a lot, your urine is concentrated, dark in colour and there is only a little of it.

Urinary tract infections

These develop when the bacteria that are usually present in the bowel pass from around the anus into the bladder through the urethra. *E. coli* is the most common bacterium involved, accounting for about 75 per cent of cases and *Proteus* species is present in many other cases.

The urethra is shorter in girls than in boys so bacteria are able to spread much more readily. As a

Urinary tract system

The kidneys filter waste products from the blood, which are excreted as urine.

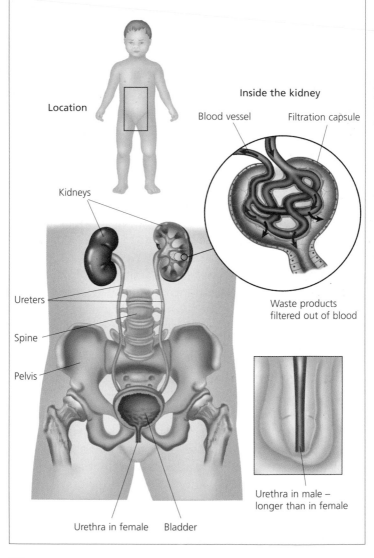

Location

Inside the kidney

Blood vessel

Filtration capsule

Kidneys

Ureters

Spine

Pelvis

Waste products filtered out of blood

Urethra in male – longer than in female

Urethra in female   Bladder

result the incidence of urinary tract infections is much higher in girls than in boys, except for children aged under three months when boys are more susceptible.

At least two per cent of boys and eight per cent of girls will have a urinary tract infection in childhood. After their first episode many of these children develop further infections over the next year or two.

Symptoms of urinary tract infections

Urinary tract infections, also known as cystitis, may be confined to the bladder, and/or affect the kidneys. In young children there will probably be no specific urinary symptoms but a child will have a raised temperature, may vomit or have diarrhoea, and may be irritable and generally unwell.

Older children may also have the above symptoms, but will have more specific urinary symptoms, such as the frequent need to pass water, a burning sensation when they do, and pain in the side or lower abdomen. The urine may have an offensive smell or be bloodstained.

Sometimes, they start day- or night-time wetting, having previously been dry. It is important to seek medical advice if a urinary tract infection is suspected because the infection may spread to the kidneys.

Testing for urinary tract infections

If a urinary tract infection is suspected your doctor will need to test the urine to see whether there is a true infection and, if so, which bacteria are responsible for it.

Your doctor will do a dipstick test on the urine, which indicates whether there is blood or protein present, but these substances can be present in other conditions so it is not a diagnostic test.

The urine can also be examined under a microscope and an instant diagnosis made. At this stage it will not be possible to say which bacteria are involved, but the urine can be sent off to the laboratory for culture and sensitivity tests to identify the cause and indicate to your doctor which is the most appropriate antibiotic.

Treatment for urinary tract infections

If any urinary tract infection is suspected and your child is under three months old, your doctor will immediately refer your child to a children's specialist for assessment and treatment.

If your child is over three months and a kidney infection is suspected your child may be referred to a children's specialist and treated with oral antibiotics; treatment can be started at once and is usually given for seven to ten days.

If your child is over three months and a lower urinary tract infection (cystitis) is suspected, your doctor may treat with oral antibiotics for three days; if your child is still unwell after 24 to 48 hours he or she will reassess your child's condition.

However, it may be necessary to change the antibiotic once results from the laboratory test identify the bacteria causing the infection. It is good practice to start treatment before the results of the tests are received because delaying the treatment can lead to the infection passing to the kidneys.

Can infections recur?

Most children make a full recovery after antibiotic treatment. However, scarring of the kidneys can occur in 5 to 15 per cent of cases. This can happen in children who have a condition known as reflux, in which urine passes backwards up the ureters towards the kidneys when the bladder is emptied. If this happens bacteria can also pass from the bladder to the kidneys, causing a kidney infection. To ascertain whether this problem exists or to see whether there is any scarring of the kidneys, special tests may be performed.

If it is thought that there is a risk of recurrent infections, a low dose of antibiotics will be given for a period of time to help prevent this happening. If medical treatment is unsuccessful and a child continues to have repeated infections, an operation may be needed to reposition the ureters so that reflux no longer occurs.

Diagnostic tests for kidney scarring or reflux

Children may have an ultrasound examination, a DMSA scan (DMSA is an abbreviation for the chemical used) or a micturating cystogram. The results from these tests are usually available after about two weeks.

Ultrasound scan

This is similar to the scan that pregnant women have. A jelly-like substance is put on the child's abdomen and a microphone-type device run over it. This device produces high-frequency sound waves and receives their echoes back to produce images of the child's kidneys on a screen. An ultrasound scan is completely painless and takes about 20 minutes.

DMSA scan

This is a very important test that allows doctors to see how well the kidneys are working and will identify whether there are any scars caused by kidney infection.

In this procedure the child is given a small injection, into a vein in the arm, of a radioactive substance called

Ultrasound scan

A device called a transducer puts out sound waves and records their returning echoes to produce pictures on a computer screen.

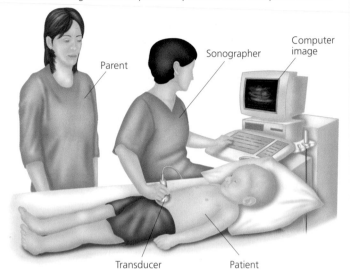

Parent

Sonographer

Computer image

Transducer

Patient

DMSA (technetium-99m-labelled dimercaptosuccinic acid or ^{99m}Tc-dimercaptosuccinic acid). This should not hurt because a local anaesthetic cream, 'magic cream', is placed over the area used for the injection. In addition there is no need to be concerned that the substance is radioactive because the amount of radiation is even less than the amount a child would receive from an X-ray.

After the injection it is necessary to wait for at least an hour for the DMSA to collect in the kidneys. Then your child needs to lie very still while a special camera, which can record the radiation emitted from the DMSA, is used to produce pictures on a monitor, which the doctor can evaluate. This takes about 10 minutes. The DMSA leaves the body quite quickly in the urine.

DMSA scan

A small amount of radioactive DMSA is injected into the patient. After about two hours the DMSA will have collected in the kidneys where images of them can be taken using a gamma camera.

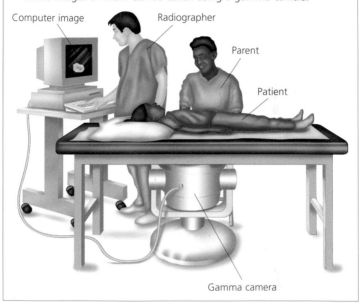

Computer image

Radiographer

Parent

Patient

Gamma camera

Micturating cystogram

This test examines the bladder and urethra. A small tube is placed into the bladder through the child's urethra. A special dye is passed through the tube, which fills the bladder. A series of X-rays are taken during the filling and emptying of the bladder in order to check for reflux (urine passing back to the kidneys).

A micturating cystogram is usually done without an anaesthetic but, if a child finds it too unpleasant, it would be postponed and carried out under a light anaesthetic.

This test tends to be reserved for certain groups of children and it may vary according to the protocol in your area. For example, in some areas it might be reserved for those children aged under one or under four who have recurrent infections.

Bedwetting

Also known as nocturnal enuresis, bedwetting is defined as an involuntary emptying, or voiding, of urine during sleep at least three times a week in a child aged five years or older. It is an extremely common problem, affecting an estimated half a million children in the UK:

- Between 15 and 20 per cent of 5 year olds
- 7 per cent of 7 year olds
- 5 per cent of 10 year olds
- 2 to 3 per cent of 12 to 14 year olds
- 1 to 2 per cent of people aged 15 and over wet their beds.

Bedwetting is twice as common in boys as in girls under the age of 10 years.

The effects of bedwetting on a child and his or her family are significant. Children can have low self-esteem and feel socially isolated. They are unable to sleep at friends' homes or go on school outings that involve overnight stays. They feel different and can be very anxious about their problem being discovered. There may also be an increased incidence of bullying.

Some parents become intolerant, believing that their child could stop wetting the bed if he or she tried harder but this is not the case. Becoming angry or punishing a child can make the situation worse.

In addition the financial burden of having a child who wets the bed is considerable and it has been calculated that it can cost several hundred pounds per year when laundry costs, and replacing bed linen and mattresses, are all taken into account.

Why does it happen?

There is no one single cause of bedwetting but it is known to be associated with several factors.

Family history

There is a definite genetic component to enuresis. If one parent wet the bed as a child, there is a 40 per cent chance that his or her own child will do it. If both parents wet their beds as children, there is a 75 per cent chance that their child will do it.

Functional bladder capacity

Children who wet their beds sometimes have small bladders, which hold a smaller volume of urine than the average. The bladder quickly becomes full and may need emptying during the night. Other children have bladders that are overactive and need to be emptied before they are full; this is described as an unstable bladder.

Nocturnal polyuria

The brain produces a hormone, arginine vasopressin (AVP), that affects urine production. Higher levels are released during the night than during the daytime; this results in decreased urine production. Studies have shown that children prone to bedwetting do not show this change in the amount of hormone released and, therefore, more urine is produced during the night than the bladder can hold.

Lack of arousal

Difficulty in waking, which is a lack of arousal from sleep, is a contributing factor to bedwetting. This does not mean, however, that enuresis is a result of deep sleep. Research has clearly shown that children who wet their bed have the same sleeping patterns as children who are not affected.

Wetting occurs throughout the sleep cycle, during both light and deep sleep, and it occurs only when the child's bladder is full and has reached its maximum capacity. Therefore, the problem lies in the child's inability to arouse or waken when their bladder is full and not in the depth of sleep.

Stress

Many parents believe, wrongly, that stress and worry are a major cause of bedwetting. If a child has been dry previously, for a period of at least six months, and then starts wetting, emotional factors may be implicated, but this is not necessarily an underlying concern in children who have never been dry at night.

Medical problem

Rarely, bedwetting can be the result of a medical problem and your doctor will detect this from the child's medical history, examination and analysis of the urine.

Treatment for bedwetting

There are a number of simple measures to help a child who is wetting the bed. If there has been no improvement after these simple measures have been tried, parents should consult their doctor, who may offer further advice and treatment or even refer the child to a specialist enuresis service:

- Parents need to be supportive, calm and encouraging.

- Don't put nappies on a older child, but you will need a good mattress protector and it is useful to use duvet and pillow protectors as well. This is particularly important for those children who produce large volumes of urine during the night.

- It is best not to lift a child and take him or her to the toilet late at night; the child will still be asleep when passing water and this is unhelpful in the long term. The child needs to be aware that he or she must wake up to go to the toilet when necessary. Also you cannot be sure that a child's functional bladder capacity has been reached at the point when he or she is woken so the brain will not be receiving messages that he or she needs to go to the toilet.

- Encourage your child to drink regularly throughout the day, but avoid fizzy drinks and those containing caffeine (tea, coffee, hot chocolate) after 6pm because they cause more urine to be produced.

- Give your child at least six or seven full drinks in a day.

- Constipation can make bedwetting worse, so it is important to try to prevent it by ensuring that children are given plenty of fruit, vegetables and cereals to eat.

- Encourage your child to take responsibility for the problem, so it is useful if the child helps change the bed and night clothes.

- Leave a light on at night or give your child a torch, so that he or she can go to the bathroom easily.

- If the bathroom is downstairs, it may be helpful to have a pot in the bedroom.
- Ensure that your child has a bath or shower every morning so that he or she does not smell of stale urine because this can result in teasing at school.

Professional treatments

If your child is referred for professional treatment there are various options: bladder re-training, enuresis alarms and medication.

Bladder re-training

This is the treatment of choice if a child has a small bladder capacity or an unstable bladder. It involves the following:

- Ensuring a regular fluid intake during the day
- Regularly going to the toilet during the day, preferably every two hours or at break time at school
- Responding immediately to any sense of wanting to pass urine
- Avoiding 'holding on' or delaying going to the toilet
- Learning to avoid hurrying when passing water because this can lead to small amounts of urine being left behind in the bladder
- Possible medication: sometimes these children also require medication to help them achieve dryness. The most commonly prescribed (by the doctor) medicine used is oxybutynin, which can be used in children aged over five years. This works by relaxing the bladder muscles and 'stabilising' the bladder. Unfortunately, side effects are quite common and

children may experience a dry mouth, constipation, nausea and stomachache.

Enuresis alarms

Alarm treatment is most useful for those children who have difficulty waking, and tends not to be used until children are at least six and often not until they are seven. Some doctors will supply alarms but they are usually distributed from specialist enuresis clinics.

The alarms work by waking the child when he or she starts to wet the bed, thus sensitising the child to respond quickly and appropriately to a full bladder during sleep. Alarm treatments have a 65 to 75 per cent success rate.

Alarms work best with children who have a normal bladder capacity and those who wet late in the night. It is also important that a child is motivated to want to stop wetting and that parents are very tolerant of the wetting because alarm treatment can disrupt the whole family.

How enuresis alarms work

There are two different basic types of alarm: a bed alarm, which is placed under the sheet, and the more commonly used body-worn alarm, which is worn under the nightclothes. They work in the same way.

For bed alarms, a special pad is put under the sheet and attached to a buzzer placed on a bedside table. For body alarms, the buzzer is pinned to a pyjama jacket, T-shirt or nightdress, and a sensor is worn between two pairs of pants or inside an absorbent disposable pad. As soon as the child starts to pass water, a buzzer is activated. The child reacts by tightening up the muscles of the pelvic floor, which stops the flow of urine, as he or she wakes up. The child is then able to go to the bathroom to finish emptying the bladder.

Enuresis alarms

There are two types of alarm: a bed alarm placed under the sheet or a body-worn device. When a child starts to pass urine the alarm is activated, waking the child who can then get up and go to the toilet.

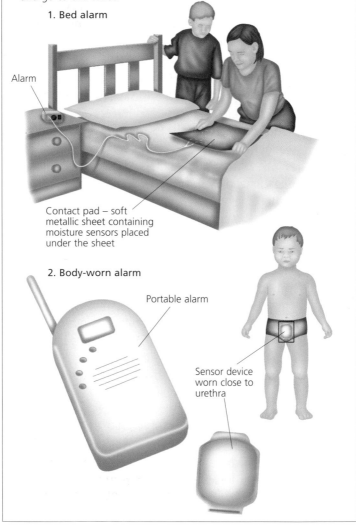

1. Bed alarm

Alarm

Contact pad – soft metallic sheet containing moisture sensors placed under the sheet

2. Body-worn alarm

Portable alarm

Sensor device worn close to urethra

The progress of treatment is closely monitored using detailed charts of the number of wet and dry nights, times at which the alarm was activated and whether the child woke to the alarm. After several weeks the child will wake automatically before the buzzer is activated or will start to sleep through the night without needing to empty the bladder.

Possible problems with alarms

They can take up to 16 weeks to be effective. If you are concerned, the doctor at the clinic or your doctor will advise on the best way forward. The following are common problems encountered with alarm treatments:

- Lack of progress – even after 16 weeks

- Not waking to the alarm

- False alarms (for example, the alarm sounding because of sweating)

- Failure of the alarm to sound

- Child not being able to stop midstream or to 'hold on' once passing water has started.

Medication for enuresis

Desmopressin, which is usually prescribed (by the doctor) as Desmotabs or Desmospray, is a synthetic version of the hormone AVP. It works by decreasing the amount of urine produced through the night. It is effective in almost 80 per cent of cases.

Medication is most successful for those children who produce large volumes of urine at night, wet infrequently and wet in the first few hours of sleep.

It can be used for as long as the wetting continues, but it is important that every three months a child has a complete treatment break for one week to see whether or not he or she has become dry spontaneously and therefore no longer requires medication.

Side effects are quite rare but it can cause headaches, stomachaches and nausea. To avoid any problems it is important for a child to decrease the amount drunk for two hours before the medication and no drinks should be allowed during the night.

When children become dry, their self-esteem increases, they feel able to participate in social activities and parents are delighted.

KEY POINTS

- Urinary tract infections are usually caused by bacteria entering the bladder from the large bowel

- Urinary tract infections can spread to the kidneys

- Some children need scans of their kidneys after urinary tract infections to check whether any scarring has occurred

- Half a million children in the UK are prone to bedwetting

- Simple measures can help bedwetting and various treatment methods are available

The skin

Conditions affecting the skin

This chapter includes conditions that affect the skin and hair, from viral and bacterial infections, such as warts or impetigo, to longer-term conditions such as eczema, and infestations such as head lice and scabies.

The anatomy of the skin

The skin is an extremely important structure with several important functions. It forms a protective barrier between the environment and the internal organs. It is a major sense organ, being able to react to touch, pressure, pain and temperature.

Pigment in the skin filters out harmful ultraviolet radiation. When exposed to cold temperatures, blood flow to the skin is reduced, helping to insulate and maintain core body temperature. When it is hot, blood flow is increased and sweating occurs to help keep the body cool.

The structure of the skin

The skin is made of three layers: epidermis, dermis and fat.
The cross-section through the skin shows the structure of these
layers and the circle shows the outer layer in more detail.
Your skin protects you against chemicals, bacteria and radiation,
helps you maintain a stable body temperature, and stops you
from losing fluid and vital body chemicals.

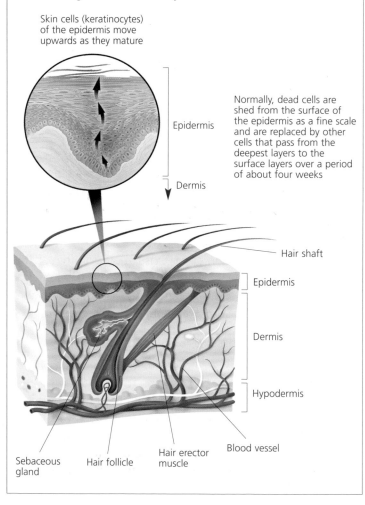

Skin cells (keratinocytes)
of the epidermis move
upwards as they mature

Epidermis

Dermis

Normally, dead cells are
shed from the surface of
the epidermis as a fine scale
and are replaced by other
cells that pass from the
deepest layers to the
surface layers over a period
of about four weeks

Hair shaft

Epidermis

Dermis

Hypodermis

Blood vessel

Hair erector
muscle

Hair follicle

Sebaceous
gland

The skin is made up of two layers:

1 The epidermis, which is the outer layer

2 The dermis, which contains blood vessels, sweat glands and nerve endings.

While the skin is intact it is also an extremely effective barrier against micro-organisms and harmful substances, but if its surface is breached in any way it can lead to superficial infections and to more serious, widespread infections.

Impetigo

This is a common bacterial infection of the skin that can affect adults as well as children. The organism responsible is *Staphylococcus* or *Streptococcus* species, which can live on the skin without causing a problem. However, if it enters the skin, usually through a cut, or an area of skin affected by eczema or a cold sore, the result can be impetigo.

Impetigo is highly infectious and spreads by direct contact with an infected person. It can also be spread through sharing towels and facecloths. Children with impetigo should not attend nursery or school until 48 hours after appropriate antibiotic treatment has begun, because it is so infectious.

Symptoms of impetigo

Impetigo begins as tiny, fluid-filled blisters, or vesicles, on the skin that rupture very easily, releasing a yellow fluid. The skin becomes red and weeping, then dries to form a honey-coloured crust. The affected area is very itchy and quite rapidly spreads to cover a large area.

Impetigo

Impetigo is caused by bacteria entering broken skin, giving rise to blistering and crusting of the skin. It often starts on the face and is most common in young children. The circle shows what it looks like.

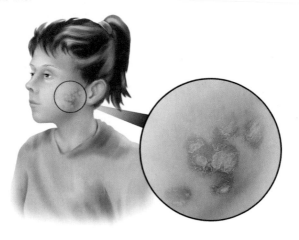

It can appear anywhere on the body but it usually appears on exposed areas of skin on the face, particularly around the mouth, hands and knees.

Treatment for impetigo

Take your child to your doctor, because impetigo may be treated with an antibiotic cream, which can be obtained only on prescription. The cream needs to be applied carefully to avoid further spread and it is important to wash your hands afterwards. Oral antibiotics are often required.

Keep an affected child's towels and facecloths separate. Tell your child not to touch the area and to wash the hands frequently.

Warts

These are caused by an extremely common, benign and usually self-limiting viral infection of the skin – the human papilloma virus, of which there are 70 different types. Warts can occur anywhere on the body but are most commonly found on the hands and feet. They probably result from the virus entering an area of damaged skin. The viruses invade skin cells and cause them to multiply, resulting in raised, rough areas, which are usually round and dotted with tiny black spots.

Plantar warts – also known as verrucas – occur on the soles of the feet; because of this they are continually under pressure from the weight of the body and, consequently, grow into the skin. These warts can be very painful.

Are warts infectious?

Spread of infection occurs by direct contact with an infected person or from contact with virus particles on flakes of skin that have been shed. Warts on the feet can be acquired from areas where people walk bare foot, for example, in communal showers and around swimming pools. If a person's immune system is suppressed – through illness, for example – he or she may develop a large number of warts.

Treatment for warts

Warts are harmless and usually disappear spontaneously as a result of natural immunity within months or years. Studies have shown that two-thirds of cases of warts disappear without treatment within a two-year period. There are many over-the-counter treatments available to treat warts if they are causing problems.

Topical treatments, those applied directly on to the wart, are often beneficial if they contain salicylic acid. Treatment is usually required daily and can last for 6 to 12 weeks. Any items that are used in this treatment, such as a pumice stone, which is used to remove the thickened skin, should be kept separate to avoid spreading the virus.

If the wart still persists after over-the-counter treatment, consult your doctor, who may offer to freeze, scrape or burn it off. Unfortunately, warts do sometimes recur. Many other different treatments have been used to treat warts but there is only very limited evidence that any of these are effective.

Molluscum contagiosum

Another viral infection of the skin, this is an infection in which shiny pimples appear, usually in clusters on the trunk and at the tops of the arms and legs. The virus is spread by close contact and is very common in children.

Symptoms

The condition begins with the appearance of one itchy, smooth, pearly white, dome-shaped spot, with a small depression at its centre.

Children tend to scratch this spot causing it to bleed, releasing viruses on to the surrounding skin so that clusters of pimples develop.

Molluscum contagiosum is a harmless infection that usually clears without treatment within 12 months.

Treatment for molluscum contagiosum

Parents are often very concerned about the appearance of this infection but it is advisable to leave the pimples alone unless they are causing distress.

Molluscum contagiosum

This is a viral infection producing multiple, shiny, pearly white pimples. The condition is harmless but very contagious.

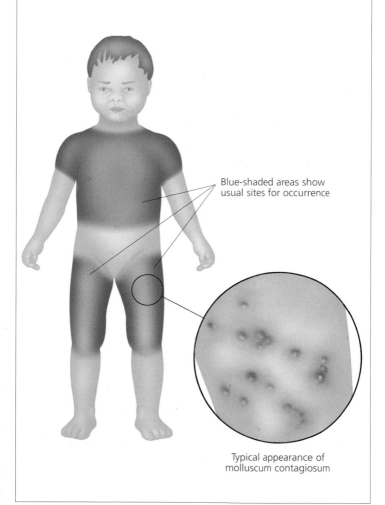

Blue-shaded areas show usual sites for occurrence

Typical appearance of molluscum contagiosum

It is important to try to avoid spread of the infection by making sure that each family member uses only his or her own towel and other such items.

Scabies

This is an infestation of the skin caused by a tiny mite called *Sarcoptes*, too small to be seen by the naked eye.

These mites are spread from person to person by close physical contact. They soon die if not kept warm and moist, so scabies is not spread by towels, bedding or clothing.

The scabies mite burrows into the skin and lays its eggs. When larvae hatch and develop into adult mites, there is an allergic response to their saliva and faeces. Typical sites of infestation are between the fingers and on the wrists. It can cause a diffuse rash on the trunk and in young children the palms of the hands and soles of the feet may be affected.

Scabies infestation is very common with an estimated 300 million cases worldwide, but it mostly affects those in less developed countries. In the developed world it is more common in institutions, in areas of social deprivation and in over-crowded homes.

Symptoms of scabies

The symptoms of scabies appear several weeks after the initial infestation and include an intense itching, which is worse at night, and a rash of pinkish-red spots or light-brown lines between the fingers (these are burrows made by the mites). The itching can occur some time before the rash appears and may persist for several weeks after successful treatment.

Scabies

Scabies is a mite infestation of the skin, causing an intensely itchy rash. The circle shows what the rash looks like and the inset shows the mite.

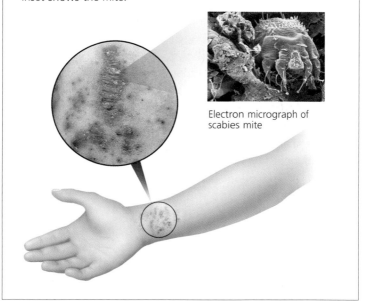

Electron micrograph of scabies mite

Diagnosis

Doctors can usually make a diagnosis by looking at the rash. To confirm diagnosis a flake of skin may be taken from one of the spots and examined under a microscope for mites. There are two forms of scabies: *classic* scabies, which affects people with a normal immune system, and *crusted* scabies, which affects people with a compromised immune system.

Treatment for scabies

Scabies is treated with a special insecticide lotion, which is applied directly to the skin. It is advised that all those living in close contact with the affected child are treated at the same time to break the chain of transmission.

The insecticide preparations available contain permethrin or malathion and your doctor or pharmacist can advise on which one to use. The lotion needs to be applied over the whole body except for the head, and left on for up to 24 hours, then washed off. One treatment may be all that is necessary, but for some lotions a repeat application is advised one week later.

Crusted scabies is much more difficult to treat and the lotion needs to be applied to the whole body, including the scalp, face and ears. In addition, a second treatment on the third day is necessary.

Eczema

This condition is especially common in children, but can affect people of any age. Eczema is an inflammation of the skin. Atopic eczema is the most common form of eczema and affects 15 to 20 per cent of children in the UK and 2 to 3 per cent of adults. Many of the children affected by it will be clear by the time they reach their teens.

The outlook for children with eczema is good with half of the children affected as babies being clear by the time they are six. Some 60 to 70 per cent of children will be clear by the time they reach their teens. However, relapses can occur in adulthood and are often related to times of stress.

Eczema tends to run in families and is closely related to asthma and hay fever. Some people have only one of these conditions, whereas others suffer from two or all three of them.

What causes eczema?

The number of children with eczema has increased substantially over the past 30 years and this is thought to be linked to environmental and lifestyle changes. Eczema is caused by a combination of a genetic predisposition to the condition and exposure to environmental allergens. These allergens include house-dust mites, feathers, animal dander, fresh-cut grass, pollens and some foods, notably cows' milk, eggs, nuts and shellfish.

Which part of the body is affected?

Atopic eczema in babies commonly affects the face, scalp and behind the ears, although in older children it is often confined to the creases of the body joints, such as behind the knees or on the insides of the elbows. It is also found on the wrists, ankles and eyelids.

Symptoms of eczema

The problem usually begins with an area of dry skin that is itchy. A child will start to scratch, which can cause the skin to become sore and inflamed. The itchiness can become even more intense and leads to further scratching. The affected skin can become blistered, weeping and crusted. Secondary infection is common.

Medical treatment for eczema

There is no cure for eczema so treatment aims to control the symptoms. The treatments range from creams, or emollients, that soften the skin to medication to control the itching.

Recognising atopic eczema

The intensely itchy rash that is characteristic of atopic eczema usually appears first in infancy. It often disappears later in childhood. The most common sites are shown, with the rash shown in more detail in the circles.

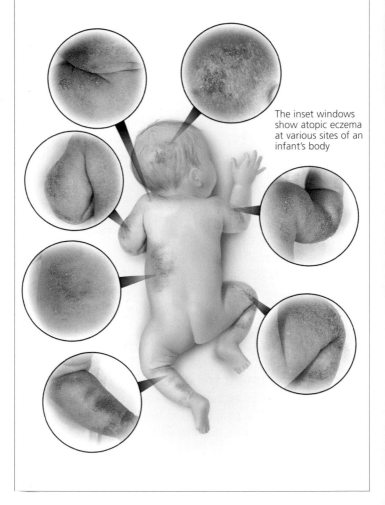

The inset windows show atopic eczema at various sites of an infant's body

The 'itch–scratch cycle'

Eczema is made worse by the 'itch–scratch cycle'. What happens is that the skin affected by eczema becomes inflamed and sore as a reaction to minor irritation. This causes the sufferer to rub and scratch the affected area, making the eczema worse. A cycle of irritation (scratching), inflammation and deterioration of the eczema sets in.

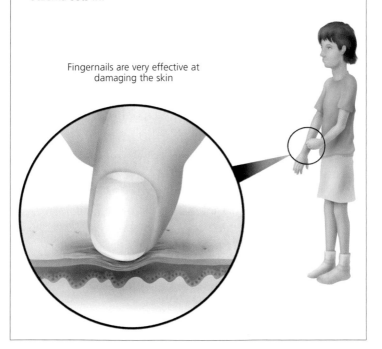

Fingernails are very effective at damaging the skin

Emollients

These are creams or oils that moisturise and protect the skin, thereby reducing inflammation and irritation.

Emollients can improve the moisture level in the skin by either preventing water loss from the skin or binding water to it. They should be used every day and there is a wide variety available. They should be used as often as necessary but at least three or four times a day is recommended to obtain maximum benefit. They are simple, safe and effective.

Emollients used to treat eczema contain no perfumes and most are lanolin free. Many can be bought over the counter at your local pharmacy or can be obtained on prescription from your doctor or health visitor.

Which emollient is best?

It is often by trial and error that you find the most suitable one:

- Ointments are used if the skin is very dry and thickened and work by holding moisture in the skin. They are very greasy and are usually applied at night.

- Creams are best for daytime use because they are easily absorbed and not as greasy or messy as ointments. They are also useful on areas of sore skin.

- Lotions are much lighter than the other kinds of moisturisers and are very easy to apply. However, they are not very effective for really dry skin.

- Bath oils not only clean the skin, lessening the risk of infection, but also leave the skin with a thin

Bath safety

A bath with lots of emollient can be dangerous because it is very slippery and people of all ages risk falling. Stop children from standing and moving around in the bath and support infants with a firm grip. Use an anti-slip mat in the bath.

Clean the bath after the use of oils because the oil causes the bath to be very slippery and can lead to an accident and injury the next time that someone uses it.

coating of oil, which traps water and helps prevent it from drying out.

Don't use ordinary soap on children with eczema, because it dries and irritates the skin. Use soap substitutes. Again it is usually by trial and error that the most suitable and most effective one is found.

Antihistamines

Medication containing an antihistamine is sometimes used to control itching but only as a short-term measure. Antihistamines make a child drowsy, which helps him or her to settle and have a more comfortable night's sleep. They should be given at least half an hour before a child goes to bed and preferably before 7pm so that they are not drowsy the next morning.

Bandages

Covering eczema with bandages should be used only when recommended by a doctor and always under medical supervision. Bandaging stops scratching and helps the skin absorb emollients. It should never be used if there are any areas of infection.

Corticosteroids

Creams containing corticosteroids are commonly used to treat eczema. They work by reducing skin inflammation. They should be applied only to inflamed areas of skin but not at the same time as the moisturiser.

Cortoicosteroid creams are very effective in reducing symptoms and within a short time of applying the cream the skin becomes less itchy and sore. The 'steroid' cream comes in varying strengths. The milder preparations are usually used as a first-line

Bath time

There is some controversy over the value of bathing a child with eczema and, if so, for how long it should last and the best additives. The following are generally accepted points on bath time:

- Child should probably not be in the bath for longer than 10–15 minutes

- Make sure that the water is not too hot because heat encourages itching, especially after a bath

- Add an emollient to the bath water in generous quantities

- If there is no obvious infection, oozing from the skin or crusting, your doctor or pharmacist may advise you to add additional antiseptic; always use as directed

- Do not use proprietary soap, bubble bath or shower gel. Use an emollient soap substitute instead and rub gently onto the skin

Hair washing
Wash your child's hair as infrequently as possible.

- When there is only moderate eczema, which does not involve the scalp, use a mild shampoo

- Wash hair separately from bath time, or at the very end of a short bath, when there is not too much emollient in the bath

- Rinse the scalp so that shampoo does not run down the body or over the face because it may irritate the skin

After the bath
Pat your child's skin dry; rubbing will provoke itching. After drying is a good time to apply emollient and other skin treatments. Apply these once the body has cooled slightly to avoid sweating under emollient.

treatment and can be bought over the counter; the stronger ones are available only on prescription. These creams are not prescribed for long-term use but are very useful for flare-ups.

Parents sometimes worry about the possible side effects of steroid creams, but, if used sparingly as directed, they are a safe and very effective treatment for eczema.

There appears to be no extra benefit from adding antibiotics to steroid creams. However, an acute flare-up is often associated with a secondary infection and this can require treatment with antibiotics.

Alternative treatments for eczema

Many people turn to alternative therapies for treatment of their eczema, especially if conventional treatments have failed. However, it is always wise to speak to your doctor before starting any of these, because he may be able to advise on reputable sources of treatment.

Chinese herbs have become a popular choice and in some cases seem to be effective. However, there have also been reported cases of liver and kidney damage so more research needs to be carried out to test their safety.

For a fuller discussion of eczema please refer to the Family Doctor Book *Understanding Eczema*.

Head lice

These are small grey–brown six-legged insects that live on, or very close to, the scalp. Infestation with head lice is very common, especially in nurseries and primary schools, with as many as four per cent (4 in 100) of children affected by them at any one time. There is some evidence to suggest that they are becoming increasingly common.

Spread by direct contact

Head lice are spread from one individual to another by direct head contact. They walk from one head to another when heads are touching. They cannot jump, fly, hop or swim. They live only on human beings so you cannot catch them from animals.

Girls are more often infected than boys. This may be a result of the fact that girls tend to spend more time with their heads in close contact and that their hair is usually longer, giving the lice more opportunity to walk from head to head. However, it is not just children who get head lice; adults (especially teachers and parents) can also be infected.

Should hair be clean and short?

Head lice have no preference for long or short hair or whether it is clean or dirty. Clean hair offers no protection but frequent washing and combing can lead to early detection and treatment.

Head lice are very difficult to see on dry hair and are difficult to detect. They vary in size from the size of a pinhead to the size of a match head. They often cause itching but this is not always the case, particularly when they have only recently infected a head. They rarely cause any other symptoms.

Life cycle of the head louse

The female louse lays eggs (commonly called 'nits') in sacs, which are firmly attached to the hair shafts. They are very small and often difficult to remove. Nits are initially dull in colour, but once hatched they are white and shiny.

The eggs hatch within 7 to 10 days and take a further 6 to 14 days to mature; they are then able to

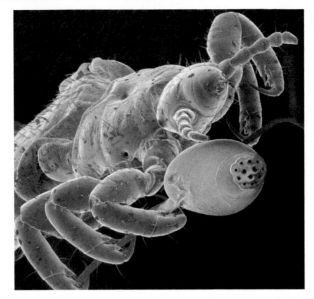

Typical appearance of a head louse under a microscope.

reproduce themselves. Immature lice tend not to move from a head until they are fully grown. They feed by biting the scalp and sucking blood from their 'host'. The life span is about three weeks. Most cases have 10 or fewer lice on the head. The lice can be present for several weeks before itching develops.

Preventing head lice

The best way to stop infection is for families to check their heads regularly, so that head lice can be found before they have a chance to multiply. They can be promptly eradicated and stopped from spreading to other family members. This is known as detection combing.

As head lice move away from a comb when the hair is dry, wash the hair first. Apply conditioner to the hair (the hair is easier to comb through and any head lice present will be more easily removed), and comb out tangles with a wide comb, then use a detection comb (see box opposite).

The whole family should be checked at the same time and treatment started if any lice are found. Chemical treatment is the only method that has been scientifically demonstrated to be effective. Everyone in the house should be checked if one person is found to have a living louse. It is also important to check other adults who have close contact with the infected child, for example, grandparents.

There is no evidence to support regular hair brushing as an avoidance technique because there is no truth in the old saying 'break its legs so it can't lay eggs'. The teacher should be informed if a child has head lice.

Tying long hair back is a sensible thing to do, although there is no direct evidence to support this being effective in avoiding head lice.

Treatment for head lice

Only begin treatment when a living, moving louse is discovered. Lotions should not be used 'just in case' because it is never a good idea to use chemicals when they are unnecessary.

- Everyone found to have living head lice must be treated at the same time, to prevent re-infection.
- Always use a head-louse lotion and not a shampoo.

Which is the most effective lotion?

There are three main groups of chemicals that are effective against head lice: pyrethroids such as phenothrin and permethrin, malathion and carbaryl.

Checking for head lice

It may take 10 to 15 minutes to check completely and thoroughly:

1 Make sure that the hair is saturated with conditioner
2 Comb out any tangles with a wide comb
3 Once the hair is completely detangled switch to a fine-toothed or detection comb

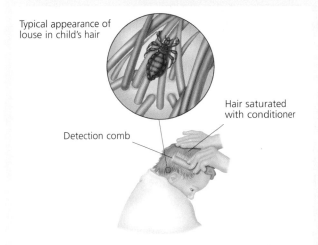

Typical appearance of louse in child's hair

Hair saturated with conditioner

Detection comb

4 Start at the base of the scalp and work up the head, working through the hair section by section
5 The teeth of the detection comb must touch the skin of the scalp, slotting into the hair roots
6 Run the comb to the ends of the hair
7 Inspect the teeth of the comb for lice after every stroke
8 Continue until you have checked the entire head
9 Repeat this procedure regularly – at least once each week to detect the presence of lice before they can spread

Carbaryl can be obtained only on prescription but the others can be bought over the counter from your pharmacist or on prescription. Whichever treatment is given, it is important to read the instructions carefully and use exactly as directed, ensuring, for example, that it is left on the hair for the correct amount of time. Some but not all lotions are capable of killing the eggs, so it is essential to check for baby lice hatching out from eggs 3 to 5 days later and again at 10 to 12 days. The lotion will need to be reapplied if any are found.

Some head lice are resistant to some of the different treatments, although there is so far only a little resistance to carbaryl. If one treatment is unsuccessful, you may need to try a different one.

Alternatives to insecticides?

Some parents are reluctant to use insecticides on their children's hair because of concerns about safety, and they seek alternative methods of treatment, such as the mechanical removal of lice with electronic combs or using head-louse repellent sprays. None of these has been scientifically proven to be effective.

Bug busting for head lice

In the 'bug-busting' method, live head lice are removed by painstakingly combing through your child's hair as described above, removing every single louse. This procedure must be repeated 4, 9 and 13 days after the initial combing to ensure that any baby lice that have hatched in the meantime are also removed.

Bug busting relies on parents being extremely thorough in removing every single louse in the hair. This is accomplished by using large amounts of conditioner so that the hair is easily untangled and lice are more easily removed.

This method cannot be advocated for the widespread treatment of lice but is a very effective way of diagnosing them and, in individual cases, if the combing is very thorough, it can be effective.

KEY POINTS

■ Impetigo is an extremely infectious skin condition that requires antibiotic treatment

■ Warts are harmless viral infections and most disappear spontaneously within two years; treatments containing salicylic acid can be useful

■ Scabies is an infestation by a particular kind of mite and is easily treated with insecticide

■ Atopic eczema affects 15 to 20 per cent of children, but 60 to 70 per cent of them will be clear of it by the time that they reach their teens

■ Head lice are spread by direct head-to-head contact. The best form of prevention is to check children's hair regularly

Rashes and infectious diseases

Common childhood infections

Young children frequently develop rashes and most of them are harmless and disappear without treatment. Many different viral and bacterial infections can cause them and some of these are described below.

When discussing common childhood infections the term 'incubation period' is often used. This refers to the time between catching the illness and becoming unwell as a result.

Chickenpox

A very common childhood infection, chickenpox is caused by the varicella-zoster virus and chiefly affects children under 10 years of age. It is spread by air-borne droplets from the upper respiratory tract of infected children, or by direct contact with the blisters. It is usually a mild illness in children but can be more serious in adults and young babies. It can be very serious in anyone who has reduced immunity, for example, those taking medication for cancer.

The incubation period for chickenpox is between 10 and 21 days but most commonly is about two weeks. Otherwise healthy children usually recover within 10 to 14 days from the onset of the rash.

Symptoms of chickenpox

The appearance of the rash is often the first sign of this infection. Many children develop very few other symptoms and may only have a mild fever and be a little unwell.

Other children become quite unwell. The rash also varies, ranging from a few spots on some children, others being covered almost from head to toe.

Chickenpox spots

Usually they appear first on the child's trunk, then the face, and finally on the arms and legs. There are commonly more spots on the trunk than anywhere else.

The spots first appear as little red dots but within a few hours they become fluid-filled blisters. The blisters are extremely fragile and easily damaged by scratching, which results because the rash is very itchy. The blisters usually dry up within a day or two and form scabs.

Chickenpox spots appear in crops over a few days and a child is infectious until the last spot scabs over. Most children recover quickly from chickenpox, but, because of the unsightly nature of the rash and to reduce the spread of infection, it is best to keep children off school for up to two weeks. Guidelines for schools state that children should be kept away from school until five days after the onset of the rash.

Chickenpox

Chickenpox is a viral infection characterised by a rash of blisters. The virus is transmitted by contact with the blisters or air-borne droplets from the coughs and sneezes of infected people.

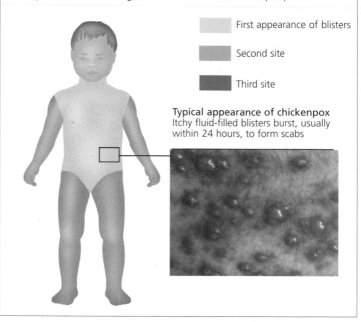

First appearance of blisters

Second site

Third site

Typical appearance of chickenpox
Itchy fluid-filled blisters burst, usually within 24 hours, to form scabs

Possible complications

Complications are rare. A secondary bacterial infection of the spots is the most common problem. It is this secondary infection that causes the spots to leave scars. Very occasionally, chickenpox leads to complications such as pneumonia, meningitis or inflammation of the heart muscle, but this is extremely rare.

Shingles and chickenpox

Once a child has had chickenpox, the varicella virus lies dormant in nerve cells. If this virus is reactivated later in life it causes a disease called shingles. The reason for the reactivation is unknown, but shingles often occurs at times of stress or other illness. The spread of this infection will cause chickenpox in someone who is not immune.

Treatment for chickenpox

In most cases no treatment is required but simple measures to reduce temperature should be used if necessary. If itching is very troublesome an antihistamine may be prescribed. If there is a secondary bacterial infection of the spots, an antibiotic may be prescribed.

Cool baths containing two tablespoons of sodium bicarbonate (bicarbonate of soda can be bought in any supermarket) can help to relieve itchiness. Calamine lotion can also help when applied to individual spots.

Mumps

This is a viral infection of the parotid (salivary) glands, which are situated below and just in front of the ears (see page 140). The virus spreads from one person to another through infected air-borne droplets by coughs or sneezes and has an incubation period of about 18 days.

The virus causes inflammation and swelling of one or both parotid glands. A child will complain of pain at the angle of the jaw on the affected side of the face. The pain is worse when eating or drinking. Children may also have a raised temperature and be generally unwell. In some instances, other salivary glands, known as submandibular glands, are also infected and pain is felt under the chin. Symptoms last for a few days.

If a boy develops mumps after puberty he has a one in four chance of developing a painful swelling of the testes known as an orchitis. This is usually confined to one side but, if both testes are involved, there is a small risk of him becoming sterile. Girls can develop a similar inflammation of the ovaries.

Other rare complications of mumps include pancreatitis (inflammation of the pancreas) and meningitis (inflammations of the layers around the brain, see page 147).

Treatment for mumps

There is no specific treatment. However, children should be given plenty of water to drink and pain relief such as paracetamol. It is best to avoid giving children

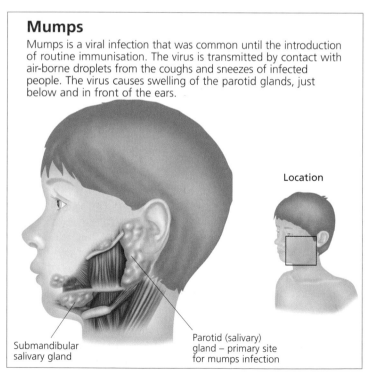

Mumps

Mumps is a viral infection that was common until the introduction of routine immunisation. The virus is transmitted by contact with air-borne droplets from the coughs and sneezes of infected people. The virus causes swelling of the parotid glands, just below and in front of the ears.

Location

Submandibular salivary gland

Parotid (salivary) gland – primary site for mumps infection

fruit juices because they increase saliva production and consequently increase the pain in the inflamed gland.

MMR vaccine

In the past mumps was very common in children but, since the introduction of an effective vaccine, the MMR (mumps, measles and rubella), it has become relatively rare. Unfortunately, over recent years the uptake of the MMR has fallen as press reports suggested a link of the vaccine to inflammatory bowel disease and autism. These links have been disproved so it is hoped that parents will again have their children immunised.

As a result of the falling numbers of children having the vaccine, there have been a number of outbreaks of mumps.

Measles

A very infectious viral illness, measles is caused by a ribonucleic acid paramyxoma virus. It has become much less common in the developed world since the introduction of the MMR immunisation. However, worldwide there are an estimated 30 million cases each year. Unfortunately, measles is still responsible for a large number of deaths in the less developed countries. The World Health Organization estimated that, in the year 2000, measles caused 770,000 deaths.

How measles spreads

The measles virus is transmitted through the air by tiny droplets produced by an infected person when he or she coughs and sneezes. The droplets can survive in the atmosphere for up to two hours in an enclosed space.

Measles most commonly occurs in the first 6 months of the year and its incubation period is 7 to 12 days.

A child with measles is infectious from one to two days before the rash appears, and up to about five days afterwards. If there are no complications children are usually well again in seven days.

Symptoms of measles

Measles usually begins in the same way as a common cold with a raised temperature, runny nose, painful, red watery eyes and a dry, hacking cough. During this stage, which usually lasts for three or four days, small white spots, known as Koplik's spots (after the man who first described them) can be seen on the inside of the child's cheeks. These are diagnostic of measles and look like small grains of salt surrounded by an area of inflammation.

After the first few days, the characteristic measles rash appears on the skin. It begins behind the ears and on the hairline, and rapidly spreads all over the body. The child's temperature may rise during this period and he or she may become more unwell.

The measles rash is a deep-red colour and single spots merge to form a distinctive blotchy appearance. The rash becomes deeper in colour and then fades into a faint brown staining after two or three days. When a child is recovering a thin layer of the skin may peel off; this is known as desquamation.

Treatment for measles

In most cases the only treatment required is rest and the recommended dose of paracetamol to bring down the temperature. A child should be given plenty of fluids. Antibiotics would be necessary only if a secondary bacterial infection developed – see below.

Measles

Measles is a highly infectious, air-borne viral disease. It mainly affects children but can occur at any age, and the adult form is usually more severe. An attack usually gives lifelong immunity.

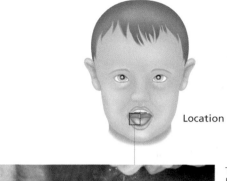

Location

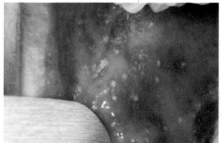

Typical appearance of Koplik's spots in measles on the inside of the cheeks. They are the early signs of measles

After three to five days a red rash appears, spreading over all the body

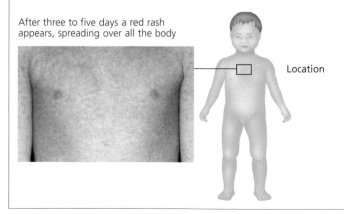

Location

Possible complications

The most common complications of measles are secondary bacterial infections of the middle ear – otitis media (see page 31), meningitis (a condition that requires urgent treatment – see page 147) and pneumonia.

A very serious complication is encephalitis, an inflammation of the brain caused by the virus. This is potentially life threatening and can have serious long-term effects, such as muscle weakness and paralysis.

Rubella

Also known as German measles, this is a mild infectious disease caused by the rubella virus. It is spread by droplet infection from the coughs and sneezes of infected people. Its incubation period is between 10 and 21 days.

This disease has become less common in the developed world because of widespread immunisation.

Symptoms of rubella

In children rubella causes little more than a rash, which begins behind the ears and on the forehead, and rapidly spreads to the trunk, arms and legs. The rash consists of tiny, flat, pink spots that last for two or three days.

A child may have a slightly raised temperature but little else. The lymph glands at the back of the neck and behind the ears can become swollen and tender, and other lymph nodes throughout the body may also be affected. Most children recover completely in 10 days.

Treatment for rubella

There is no specific treatment. It is necessary only to give plenty of fluids and, if a child has a temperature,

Rubella (German measles)

Rubella, also called German measles, usually causes little more than a mild rash. However, it can cause serious birth defects in a fetus if the mother contracts the disease in early pregnancy.

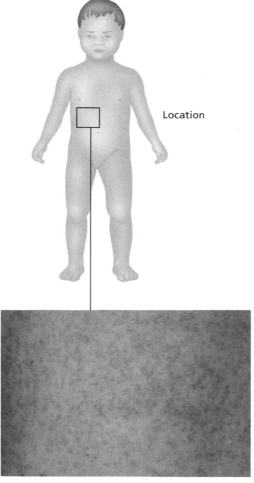

Location

Typical appearance of rubellar rash

you can give him or her paracetamol to reduce the fever. Children usually make a full and rapid recovery.

Possible complications

The only very rare complication is a temporary inflammation of many different joints, which causes pain and swelling and is known as a polyarthritis.

Rubella in pregnancy

The rubella virus is extremely serious if caught by a woman when she is in the early stages of pregnancy.

The fetus can be very badly affected and the baby can be born with a number of different abnormalities; he or she could be blind, deaf, or have a congenital heart disease or a learning disability.

It is vital, therefore, that any child with rubella be kept well away from women who are pregnant or who are hoping to become so.

Women can be tested

One attack of rubella gives lifelong immunity, so once a child has had it he or she will never be affected again. However, in common with other 'nevers' in medicine there are a few exceptions.

A woman can protect herself and her planned baby against rubella by having a blood test to find out whether or not she has rubella antibodies.

If she does not have clear evidence of immunity she should be given a rubella immunisation before she becomes pregnant and avoid becoming pregnant for one month. This cautious approach is the one recommended by the experts.

Meningitis

This is one of the most serious infections of childhood and probably causes more anxiety for parents than any other illness. Meningitis is an inflammation of a special lining that surrounds the brain and spinal cord known as the meninges.

Anyone can develop meningitis but certain groups of people are most at risk and these are:

- Children aged under five
- Teenagers
- Young adults
- Elderly people.

Meningitis is most commonly caused by either viruses or bacteria, but may be the result of other parasites in the tropics.

Viral meningitis

This type of meningitis is more common than bacterial meningitis and is far less serious. It is most common in young adults and can be caused by a variety of different viruses.

The most common viruses involved are Coxsackie virus and echoviruses, but meningitis can also be a complication of measles, polio, herpes simplex and chickenpox. It is spread by coughing and sneezing or through poor hygiene, for example, not washing the hands after going to the toilet. The incubation period for viral meningitis can be up to three weeks.

Treatment for viral meningitis

Antibiotics cannot combat viruses (see page 8) and so treatment usually consists of good nursing care. A full recovery is usual and most children are well again in two weeks. However, viral meningitis can leave an individual feeling tired and sometimes depressed for weeks or even months.

Bacterial meningitis

This type of meningitis is fairly uncommon but is potentially life threatening. In the UK the two main bacteria that cause it are meningococci and pneumococci.

In the past another bacterium, *Haemophilus influenzae* type b, caused about two-fifths of bacterial meningitis cases; however, since the introduction of Hib immunisation in 1992 this has become uncommon.

Immunisation programme for meningitis

Hib immunisation is given to babies in three doses when they are two, three and four months old with a booster at twelve months. There are various groups of meningococcal bacteria: A, B, C, W135 and Y.

Groups A and Y rarely cause disease in the UK, whereas group B causes the highest number of cases. At present there is no effective vaccine against group B, but scientists are developing this and it should be available in the future.

Immunisation against group C was introduced in November 1999 and is now given in three separate doses as part of the routine childhood immunisation programme. Group W135 has caused only a small number of cases. Immunisation against pneumoccocal disease was introduced in 2006; the vaccine is given as two doses at two and four months with a booster around thirteen months.

Is bacterial meningitis infectious?

Most cases of meningitis are isolated and not related to other cases. The risk of catching meningitis from someone whom you meet is very small. The risk is slightly higher if you are living in the same household.

The meningococcal and pneumococcal bacteria are both very common and live naturally in the back of the nose and throat. Being a carrier of these bacteria can boost immunity and, at any one time, between 10 and 25 per cent of the population are carriers of the meningococcal bacteria.

The bacteria are spread by coughing, sneezing and kissing. These bacteria cannot live for long outside the body, so they cannot be picked up from water, swimming pools or buildings. A person can carry the bacteria without developing meningitis. Only occasionally do the bacteria overcome the body's defences and cause the disease.

The incubation period for bacterial meningitis is between 2 and 10 days. It may take several weeks or even months for a full recovery from this illness.

Septicaemia in meningitis

If the bacteria enter the bloodstream and start multiplying they cause blood poisoning. This is known as meningococcal septicaemia and is extremely serious. The increasing numbers of bacteria release toxins or poisons into the bloodstream and these can damage blood vessels and any organ in the body.

Patients with septicaemia often, but not always, develop a characteristic rash: this can start anywhere on the body and initially looks like tiny blood spots that gradually increase in size and, eventually, form areas that look like bruises. To assess whether the rash is

Signs and symptoms of meningitis

One of the most worrying things about meningitis is how difficult it can be to diagnose, because the initial symptoms can be very similar to those of flu. They can sometimes develop over one or two days and, in other cases, within a few hours. Symptoms do not develop in any particular order and some may not appear at all. There are some differences in the symptoms in babies to those in older children and adults.

Symptoms in babies
- High temperature, fever, possibly with cold hands and feet
- Vomiting or refusing feeds
- High-pitched, moaning, whimpering cry
- Blank, staring expression
- Pale, blotchy complexion
- Arched back and retraction of neck (head forced back)
- Baby may be floppy, dislike being handled and be fretful
- Baby is difficult to wake or lethargic
- The fontanelle (soft spot on baby's head) may be tense or bulging
- Possible distinctive purple rash, caused by septicaemia

Symptoms in children and adults
- High temperature, fever, possibly with cold hands and feet
- Vomiting, sometimes diarrhoea
- Severe headache
- Neck stiffness (unable to touch the chin to the chest)
- Joint or muscle pains, sometimes stomach cramps with septicaemia
- Dislike of bright lights
- Drowsiness
- Fits
- The person may be confused or disoriented
- Possible distinctive purple rash, caused by septicaemia

CALL OUT YOUR DOCTOR
If your child shows any of the symptoms listed, call your doctor. Do not to wait for the rash to appear; this may be the last symptom to appear and in many cases may not appear at all.

Glass test

Press the side of a clear glass firmly against the spots. If it is a septicaemia rash, the spots will not fade. The rash is harder to see on dark skin but is most apparent on the paler areas of skin such as the palms of the hands or the soles of the feet.

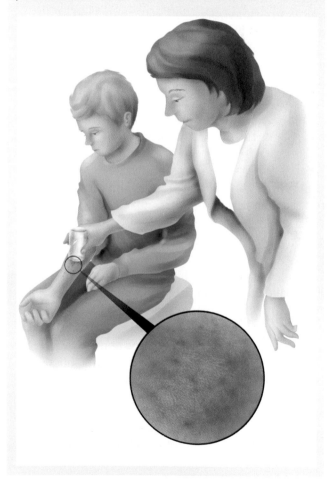

septicaemia, the glass test can be carried out (see box on page 151).

Long-term outlook

After septicaemia patients may need skin grafts or even have affected limbs, fingers or toes amputated. Bacterial meningitis is fatal in one in ten cases, and one in seven survivors is left with some kind of disability such as deafness, epilepsy or brain damage.

Meningitis can also lead to other long-term problems, such as general tiredness, behavioural problems, children forgetting skills that may only recently have been acquired, headaches and sleep disturbance. All these symptoms will improve with time and parents need to be patient and understanding.

Treatment for bacterial meningitis

Urgent treatment with antibiotics and appropriate hospital management are essential for anyone with this disease. The sooner treatment is initiated the greater the chance of a full recovery. If there is a delay in contacting your doctor, call an ambulance.

Preventing spread of meningitis

Apart from vaccines there is no known way to protect against meningitis. However, it is not highly infectious and only the patient's close friends and family contacts are at significant risk of becoming ill. Antibiotics will be offered to everyone living and sleeping in the same household as the affected person, and to those who have intimately kissed the infected person, but others, such as school friends or colleagues, do not normally need treatment.

The most important aspect of prevention is raising awareness of the signs and symptoms of the disease and being prepared to take immediate action.

It is now known that children living in a household in which people smoke have an increased chance of contracting meningitis.

The Meningitis Trust

This is an organisation that offers support for patients, families and friends affected by meningitis. They provide education to help health-care professionals and the general public to identify meningitis. They also fund research into vaccines and improved treatments for the disease and the after effects. They offer a 24-hour helpline and their contact telephone number is at the end of this book.

KEY POINTS

- Many different infections cause a rash

- The incubation period is the time between catching the illness and becoming unwell

- Mumps is a viral infection of the parotid salivary gland

- The number of cases of mumps in the UK is increasing and decreasing numbers of children are having the MMR immunisation

- It is very important that all children have the measles, mumps and rubella (MMR) immunisation

- Meningitis is one of the most serious infections of childhood but its symptoms do not develop in any particular order

- If you suspect that your child has meningitis, do not wait for the rash to appear because this may be the last and most serious symptom to develop; if at all worried parents must obtain urgent medical advice

Prevention is better than cure

This saying, 'Prevention is better than cure', is based on the best possible advice. But you cannot always prevent a child having the occasional cough or cold or, in some cases, developing a more serious illness.

However, without doubt, you can decrease the number of infections that both children and adults develop by living healthier lifestyles and taking the necessary preventive measures that are available, for example, making sure that your child's immunisation programme is completed.

Eat a healthy diet

Making the right food choices is one of the important ways to feel and remain healthier. Eating healthily yourself is the best way to encourage children to develop good eating habits.

Giving a child the right balance of foods will give them all the nutrients that they need for growth and development, and will also help reduce the risk of serious disease later in life. General principles of eating healthily include the following:

- Eat at regular intervals
- Eat plenty of fruit and vegetables – at least five portions a day
- Avoid eating too many salty and sugary foods
- Eat fewer fatty foods
- No alcohol for children and decreasing alcohol intake in adults
- Drink plenty of water
- Eat meals that contain a mix of the recognised food groups, and vitamins and minerals.

The main food groups

Group 1: carbohydrates

These are foods such as bread, cereals and potatoes. A food from this group should be eaten at every meal and should cover about a third of the plate. They are filling, low in fat and provide natural energy.

Group 2: fruit and vegetables

It is recommended that you eat at least five portions each day. Prolonged cooking destroys vitamins and therefore vegetables need to be eaten raw, or cooked as quickly as possible in as little water as possible. Steaming, poaching and using the microwave are all ideal cooking methods.

Group 3: proteins

These are found in meat, fish, eggs, beans and pulses. Two small portions of these each day are usually sufficient.

Group 4: dairy products

Although adults need to reduce their fat intake, young children should not. It is important to remember that children aged under two years should be given full-cream milk, and not skimmed or semi-skimmed milk as recommended for adults. If a child aged under five has a poor diet it is recommended that he or she continues to have full-cream milk.

Group 5: foods that contain fat and sugar

It is the food in this group – crisps, biscuits, cake, pastries and fat spreads – that you should eat as little of as possible.

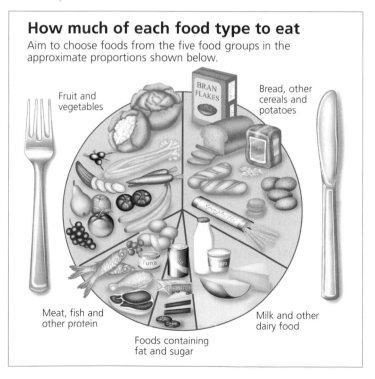

How much of each food type to eat

Aim to choose foods from the five food groups in the approximate proportions shown below.

Fruit and vegetables

Bread, other cereals and potatoes

Meat, fish and other protein

Foods containing fat and sugar

Milk and other dairy food

Regular exercise

Getting plenty of exercise is the next most important requirement, after eating healthily, if families are to remain fit and well.

Exercise is particularly good if it is taken outside in the fresh air. Many children spend an excessive amount of time sitting down, watching television and videos or playing computer games, and spend very limited amounts of time running around outside. This is thought to be responsible in part for the rising numbers of obese children.

Inactivity is now believed to be the most important threat to general health. Exercise options for children include the following:

- Walking to and from school
- Walking in the local park
- Walking to and from the shops/supermarket
- Swimming regularly, perhaps with a group of friends
- Cycling in the garden or local park
- Organised team sports such as football or with the child's friends from nursery or school
- Organised children's classes such as dance, yoga, gymnastics, martial arts.

Plenty of sleep

It is vital for young children to have regular bedtime routines and plenty of sleep. The number of hours that a child needs to sleep vary but, in general:

- Newborn babies sleep for 16.5 hours a day

- Two- to three-month-old babies sleep for 15 hours a day
- Six-month-old babies sleep 14.25 hours a day
- Twelve-month-old babies sleep 13.75 hours a day
- Two-year-old children are asleep 13 hours a day.

These are averages and children are all different; it is important, however, that parents ensure that their children have an adequate amount of sleep and go to bed early rather than late.

This enhances a child's ability to thrive mentally, emotionally and physically, to fight off infection and illness, to enjoy their daily life and to develop to their fullest potential.

Hygiene in the home

Preventing the spread of germs and illness depends on following a good level of hygiene in your home, being strict about hand-washing routines, especially after going to the toilet and before eating, and regular bathing.

It is extremely important not to smoke around children because smoking increases the child's risk of ear and chest infections. It also increases the risk of sudden infant death syndrome or a cot death (see box overleaf).

Home safety – accident prevention

Providing a safe environment within the home is very important. Accidents in the home are the major cause of injury in young children. Poisoning, falls and drowning are the most common accidents. Every item that has the potential to harm, for example, bleach, medicines and matches, should be locked away. Safety gates, fireguards

Sudden infant death syndrome (SIDS)

This is the sudden and unexpected death of an infant under the age of one year and for which no cause can be found, even after reviewing the medical history, examination of the scene of the death and *post mortem*. It is also known as cot death because it usually occurs when a seemingly healthy baby is put to bed and is then later found dead.

Reducing the risk of cot death

The incidence of sudden infant deaths has been declining over the past ten years. Although the cause of these deaths is unknown studies have highlighted a number of risk factors. By following some simple advice the risk of cot death can be reduced:

- Place your baby on his or her back to go to sleep.

- Stop smoking during pregnancy: the less you smoke, the lower the risk.

- Do not allow anyone to smoke in the same room as your baby and do not take your baby into smoky places.

- Do not let your baby get too hot. In summer your baby may need only a sheet to cover him or her. In winter two or three blankets may be all that is necessary. Do not use duvets, quilts, baby nests or pillows. Babies do not need hot rooms. About 18°C is comfortable.

- When you put a baby to bed, his or her head should be uncovered and the feet should be placed

Sudden infant death syndrome (SIDS) (contd)

at the foot of the cot. This prevents a baby from wriggling down under the covers.

- It is best for babies to sleep in their own cots, not your bed. There is a link between sharing a bed and cot death if you or your partner is a smoker, has recently drunk alcohol, has taken drugs or medication to help sleep, or is very tired.

- If your baby is unwell seek medical advice promptly.

- The safest place for your baby to sleep is in a cot in your room for the first six months.

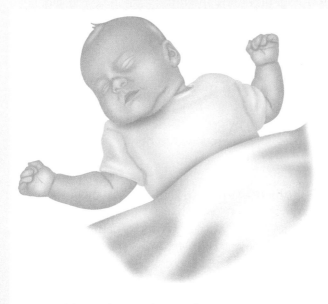

Sleep safely – make sure that you follow the guidelines when putting your baby in his or her cot.

and plug socket covers should all be used. Minor accidents cannot always be prevented but it is possible to minimise them by taking these simple precautions.

Your child's immunisation schedule

Keeping up to date with a child's immunisations is of paramount importance. This is the safest and most effective way of protecting children against serious illnesses and infections.

Immunisation is a way of boosting the body's defences against infections with which the child may come into contact in the future. Injecting a vaccine, which contains an altered, or inactivated, form of the infected agent, brings about this immunity. The vaccine stimulates the body to produce antibodies against the disease so that, if the child is exposed to the organism in the future, he or she is protected against it.

How vaccines are given

Most vaccines are given by injection although a few, such as polio, can be given orally. For most immunisations several injections are required to obtain complete protection from the disease.

Main immunisations

During childhood children should be protected against tetanus, diphtheria, whooping cough (pertussis), polio, meningitis C, *Haemophilus influenzae* type b (Hib), measles, mumps, rubella and pneumococcal infection.

The schedule of routine immunisations has changed many times in the past and the most recent significant change took place in September 2006. Be sure to check your child's immunisation schedule with your doctor and health visitor.

Risks of immunisation

Immunisations have few side effects. There may be inflammation around the injection site and a lump may develop but this is nothing to worry about. A child may also have a mild fever and be slightly unwell.

Rarely, a child may have an allergic reaction, but the health professionals giving the injections are aware of the signs and symptoms of this and are trained to treat such a reaction immediately.

The risks to children from routine immunisations are much lower than the risks associated with the actual diseases.

There are very few reasons for a child not to be immunised. The major reasons not to give immunisation are when a child has any of the following because they may affect the immune system:

- The child has a high temperature on the day of the immunisation.

- The child is receiving treatment for cancer.

- The child has a current illness and is taking medication.

Foreign travel

Prevention is better than cure, in no context more so than that of foreign travel. Travelling abroad, outside Europe, may demand an immunisation programme for both children and their parents. This needs to be organised well ahead of the trip because some vaccines, such as that for typhoid, take a month or more to become active in the body and others require more than one injection.

Recommended immunisation schedule

When to immunise	Diseases protected against
2 months	Diphtheria, tetanus, pertussis (whooping cough), polio and Hib, pneumococcal infection
3 months	Diphtheria, tetanus, pertussis, polio and Hib, meningitis C
4 months	Diphtheria, tetanus, pertussis, polio and Hib, meningitis C, pneumococcal infection
12 months	Hib and meningitis C
13 months	Measles, mumps and rubella, pneumococcal infection
3 years 4 months to 5 years	Diphtheria, tetanus, pertussis, polio, measles, mumps and rubella
13–18 years	Tetanus, diphtheria and polio

Check local immunisation requirements

You should check that the area that you are going to visit is safe for diseases such as polio, diphtheria, tetanus, hepatitis, typhoid, cholera, yellow fever and malaria. Your doctor's surgery will have information about the current medical requirements and recommendations for the region that you are visiting. Immunisation and/or medication is available for most tropical diseases either from or through the family doctor.

Recommended immunisation schedule (contd)

Vaccine given

DTaP/IPV/Hib and pneumococcal conjugate vaccine (PCV)

DTaP/IPV/Hib and MenC

DTaP/IPV/Hib, MenC and PCV

Hib/MenC

MMR and PCV

DTap (high-strength diphtheria, tetanus and acellular pertussis)/IPV or dTap (low-strength diphtheria, tetanus and acellular pertussis)/IPV and MMR

Td (tetanus and low-strength diphtheria)/IPV

Long journeys
If you travel by air, take boiled sweets for your child to help with pressure earache. To help with the boredom of long journeys, take plenty of distractions in the form of games and books.

Illness while abroad
Upset stomach, food poisoning and gastroenteritis all demand medical attention if the symptoms persist for more than 24 hours and plenty of fluids, principally

water (see page 90). Do not give colas or sweetened fruit juices, such as clear apple juice, because this will intensify the symptoms and delay recovery.

Use bottled water unless you are certain that the local water is clean.

KEY POINTS

■ Providing a well-balanced diet is an important way to ensure that children remain healthy

■ Plenty of exercise and having good sleep routines are also important

■ Keeping up to date with a child's immunisations is of great importance

■ Check immunisation requirements before you travel

■ The incidence of sudden infant death has been decreasing over the past 10 years since new advice has been given

Contents of a family medicine box

It is useful to have a supply of frequently used medicines and first-aid items at home. It is also useful to take items with you on holiday and keep a basic first-aid kit in your car.

It is important, however, to observe a few important rules:

- All medicines should be kept in a locked container out of the reach of children.

- Never use medicines that are past their expiry date.

- Always read the instructions carefully and give the correct dose for the age of the individual needing them.

- Always dispose of out-of-date medicines correctly by taking them to your local or hospital pharmacy. Never put them in the rubbish or flush them down the toilet.

- If your child has to take regular medication, ensure that you keep sufficient spares, so that you won't run out.

Family medicines
Medicine box

A home medicine box should contain the following items:

- Simple painkillers such as paracetamol or ibuprofen, and dosing measure (oral syringe or spoon)
- Oral rehydration fluid sachet such as Dioralyte
- Anti-diarrhoeal medicines (for adults only)
- Laxatives
- Thermometer – ideally digital or strip
- Antacid indigestion remedies.

First aid box

- Plasters
- Roller bandages – either gauze or crêpe
- Small and large sterile dressing
- Triangular bandages
- Disposable gloves
- Scissors, tweezers and safety pins
- Antiseptic cream
- It may also useful to have sun screen, travel sickness tablets, antihistamines, sunburn treatment and an eye wash in your box.

Useful addresses

Where can I find out more?

We have included the following organisations because, on preliminary investigation, they may be of use to the reader. However, we do not have first-hand experience of each organisation and so cannot guarantee the organisation's integrity. The reader must therefore exercise his or her own discretion and judgement when making further enquiries.

General information

Benefits Enquiry Line

Tel: 0800 882200

Minicom: 0800 243355

Website: www.dwp.gov.uk

N. Ireland: 0800 220674

Government agency giving information and advice on sickness and disability benefits for people with disabilities and their carers.

Citizens Advice Bureau

Myddelton House, 115–123 Pentonville Road
London N1 9LZ
Tel: 020 7833 2181
Website: www.adviceguide.org.uk

HQ of national charity offering a wide variety of
practical, financial and legal advice. Network of local
centres throughout the UK can be found in the phone
book.

Clinical Knowledge Summaries

Sowerby Centre for Health Informatics at Newcastle
(SCHIN Ltd), Bede House, All Saints Business Centre
Newcastle upon Tyne NE1 2ES
Tel: 0191 243 6100
Website: www.cks.library.nhs.uk

A website mainly for GPs giving information for patients
listed by disease plus named self-help organisations.

Great Ormond Street Hospital for Children NHS Trust

Great Ormond Street
London WC1N 3JH
Tel: 020 7609 1871
Website: www.ich.ucl.ac.uk

Produces information leaflets on childhood diseases,
jointly compiled with the Institute of Child Health.
They are available from the Institute of Child Health's
website: www.ich.ucl.ac.uk/factsheets. Or they can be
requested by telephoning 020 7829 7862.

Meningitis Trust
Fern House, Bath Road
Stroud GL5 3TJ
Tel: 01453 768000
Helpline: 0800 028 1828 (24 hours a day)
Website: www.meningitis-trust.org.uk

National Institute for Health and Clinical Excellence (NICE)
MidCity Place, 71 High Holborn
London WC1V 6NA
Tel: 020 7067 5800
Website: www.nice.org.uk

Provides national guidance on the promotion of good health and the prevention and treatment of ill-health. Patient information leaflets are available for each piece of guidance issued.

NSPCC (National Society for the Prevention of Cruelty to Children)
42 Curtain Road
London EC2A 3NH
Tel: 020 7825 2500 (admin)
Tel: 020 7825 2775 (information)
Child protection helpline: 0808 800 5000
Textphone: 0800 056 0566
Website: www.nspcc.org.uk

Provides information (also in Welsh and five Asian languages), advice and counselling to anyone concerned about a child's safety. Carries out research and campaigns on behalf of children. Liaises with other agencies and offers training courses for parents and professionals through 180 community-based projects in England, Wales and Northern Ireland.

Open University
PO Box 724
Milton Keynes MK7 6ZS

Tel: 01908 653231
Website: www.open.ac.uk

The Faculty of Health and Social Care produces home study packs and videos on babies, children, teenagers and being a parent, which you can use individually or in groups.

Parentline Plus (merged with Parent Network)
520 Highgate Studios, 53–79 Highgate Road, Kentish Town
London NW5 1TL
Tel: 020 7284 5500
Helpline: 0808 800 2222
Textphone: 0800 783 6783
Website: www.parentlineplus.org.uk

For parents under stress nationally. Provides general confidential information and runs parenting courses. Accepts referrals via Social Services.

Specific information

ADHD
ADDISS Attention Deficit Information Services
Premier House, 112 Station Road, Edgware
London HA8 7BJ

Tel: 020 8952 2800
Website: www.addiss.co.uk

Provides information, support and training. Can refer to local groups in the UK. Mail order catalogue for publications sent on request.

Allergy
Allergy UK (British Allergy Foundation)
3 White Oak Square, London Road
Swanley, Kent BR8 7AG
Tel: 01322 619864
Helpline: 01322 619898
Website: www.allergyuk.org
Chemical sensitivity helpline: 01322 619898

Encompasses all types of allergies and offers information, quarterly newsletter and support network; translation cards for travel abroad. Funds research. Annual subscription £15.

Anaphylaxis Campaign
PO Box 275, Farnborough
Hants GU14 6SX
Tel: 01252 373793
Helpline: 01252 542029
Website: www.anaphylaxis.org.uk

Campaigns for better awareness of life-threatening allergic reactions from food and drug allergies to bee and wasp stings. Produces a wide range of educational newssheets and videos and has extensive support network. Send an SAE for information.

Asthma
Asthma UK
Summit House, 70 Wilson Street
London EC2A 2DB
Tel: 020 7786 4900
Helpline: 0845 701 0203
Website: www.asthma.org.uk

Provides a wide range of information and support for
people with asthma and their families. Helpline staffed
by specialist asthma nurses. Has local support groups
and funds medical research. Offers special supervised
activity holidays for young people with asthma and/or
eczema.

Asthma UK Scotland
4 North Charlotte Street
Edinburgh EH2 1JE
Tel: 0131 226 2544
Helpline: 0845 701 0203
Website: www.asthma.org.uk

Funds research and offers a range of information
about coping with asthma. Helpline staffed by
specialist asthma nurses. Has local support groups.
Offers special supervised activity holidays for young
people with asthma and/or eczema.

British Lung Foundation
73–75 Goswell Road
London EC1V 7ER
Tel: 020 7688 5555
Helpline: 0845 850 5020
Website: www.lunguk.org

Raises funds for research into all forms of lung disease. Offers information leaflets and has a series of self-help groups around the country, the Breathe Easy Club, largely run by patients.

Bedwetting and soiling
ERIC (Enuresis Resource and Information Centre)
34 Old School House, Britannia Road, Kingswood
Bristol BS15 8DB
Tel: 0117 960 3060 (Mon–Fri 10am–4pm)
Helpline: 0845 370 8008
Website: www.eric.org.uk

Offers information leaflets and advice about enuresis and encopresis; sells bedwetting protection and alarms, and also resource materials for professionals.

Dyslexia
British Dyslexia Association
98 London Road
Reading RG1 5AU
Tel: 0118 966 2677
Helpline: 0118 966 8271
Website: www.bda-dyslexia.org.uk

Raises awareness of dyslexia; provides advice, local contact and resources.

The Dyslexia Institute
Park House, Wick Road
Egham, Surrey TW20 0HH
Tel: 01784 222300
Website: www.dyslexia-inst.org.uk

Provides information, assessment and teaching of people with dyslexia and the training of teachers.

Dyspraxia
Dyscovery Centre
University of Wales, Allt-yr-yn Campus
Newport NP20 5DA
Tel: 01633 432330
Website: www.dyscovery.co.uk

Private assessment centre for neurodevelopmental problems, providing information and training for children and adults with living and learning difficulties.

Dyspraxia Foundation
8 West Alley, Hitchin
Herts SG5 1EG
Tel: 01462 455016
Helpline: 01462 454986
Website: www.dyspraxiafoundation.org.uk

Offers information and support via UK network to parents and professionals. Arranges conferences for parents, carers and professionals.

Ears
British Academy of Audiology
PO Box 346
Peterborough PE6 7EG
Tel: 01733 253976
Website: www.baaudiology.org

Deafness Research UK
330–332 Gray's Inn Road

London WC1X 8EE
Voice: 020 7833 1733
Text: 020 7915 1412
Website: www.deafnessresearch.org.uk

The only UK charity dedicated to funding medical research into hearing impairment. Offers information service on hearing-related illnesses.

National Deaf Children's Society (NDCS)
15 Dufferin Street
London EC1Y 8UR
Tel: 020 7490 8656
Helpline: 0808 800 8880
Website: www.ndcs.org.uk

Eyes
LOOK, National Federation of Families with Visually Impaired Children
c/o Queen Alexandra College, 49 Court Oak Road, Harborne
Birmingham B17 9TG
Tel: 0121 428 5038
Website: www.look-uk.org

Offers information, help and support for parents who have visually impaired children; access to benefits, education and grants.

Royal College of Ophthalmologists
17 Cornwall Terrace
London NW1 4QW
Tel: 020 7935 0702
Website: www.rcophth.ac.uk

Professional college for eye specialists that produces a number of leaflets about a variety of eye diseases.

Skin Problems

British Association of Dermatologists and British Dermatological Nursing Group
4 Fitzroy Square
London W1T 5HQ
Tel: 020 7383 0266
Website: www.bad.org.uk

Information on a range of skin diseases, including eczema. Provides members of the public with a list of dermatologists in their area, but does not recommend specific doctors. To consult a dermatologist, it is necessary to be referred by a GP.

National Eczema Society
Hill House, Highgate Hill
London N19 5NA
Tel: 020 7281 3553
Helpline: 0870 241 3604 (Mon–Fri 8am–8pm)
Website: www.eczema.org

Provides a wide range of information leaflets for eczema sufferers, their carers and health professionals.

The Psoriasis Association
Dick Coles House, 2 Queensbridge
Northampton NN4 7BF
Tel: 01604 251620
Helpline: 0845 676 0076
Website: www.psoriasis-association.org.uk

This organisation provides information on different aspects of psoriasis, as well as promoting research. It produces a journal four times a year and organises an annual conference on psoriasis.

Special educational needs
Advisory Centre for Education
Unit 1C, Aberdeen Studios, 22 Highbury Grove
London N5 2DQ
Tel: 020 7704 3370
Helpline: 0808 800 5793 (Mon–Fri 10am–5pm)
Order line: 020 7704 9822 for Exclusion Pack
Website: www.ace-ed.org.uk

Independent national advice centre for parents of children in state schools. Offers information and advice on the law and school issues. Also offers training.

For parents with babies and young children
Association for Post Natal Illness
145 Dawes Road, Fulham
London SW6 7EB
Helpline: 020 7386 0868 (Mon, Wed, Fri 10am–2pm; Tues, Thurs 10am–5pm)
Website: www.apni.org

Provides information leaflets and support to health professionals and anyone involved with postnatal depression. Can refer to mothers who have recovered from postnatal depression.

Cry-sis Helpline and Support Group
BM Cry-sis
London WC1N 3XX
Helpline: 0845 122 8669
Website: www.cry-sis.org.uk

Contact this organisation if you think your baby cries
excessively. Cry-sis provides local support groups,
newsletters and publications.

Family Welfare Association
501–505 Kingsland Road
London E8 4AU
Tel: 020 7254 6251
Website: www.fwa.org.uk

Runs centres that provide home support, drop-ins,
group discussions, and training courses for parents
with babies and toddlers in the London area.

Home-Start
2 Salisbury Road
Leicester LE1 7QR
Tel: 0116 233 9955
Helpline: 0800 068 6368
Website: www.home-start.org.uk

Offers information leaflets and parent-to-parent
support in your own home in the UK and to British
Forces overseas. Provides training to volunteers.

Meet-A-Mum Association (MAMA)

7 Southcourt Road, Linslade
Leighton Buzzard, Beds LU7 2QF
Tel: 0845 120 6162
Postnatal depression helpline: 0845 120 3746 (7–10pm)
Website: www.mama.co.uk

Local social gatherings and mum-to-mum contact for
mums who are depressed postnatally or feel exhausted
and isolated after the birth.

National Childbirth Trust

Alexandra House, Oldham Terrace
Acton W3 6NH
Tel: 0870 770 3236
Breast-feeding helpline: 0870 444 8708 (8am–10pm)
Website: www.nctpregnancyandbabycare.com

Provides antenatal and postnatal support, information
on childbirth and parenting and useful leaflets. Pre-
and postnatal classes and breast-feeding counselling by
trained teachers.

National Childminding Association

Royal Court, 81 Tweedy Road
Bromley, Kent BR1 1TW
Tel: 020 8464 6164
Helpline: 0845 880 0044
Website: www.ncma.org.uk

Promotes registered childminding in England and
Wales and provides training.

Pre-School Learning Alliance
The Fitzpatrick Building, 188 York Way
London N7 9AD
Tel: 020 7697 2500
Website: www.pre-school.org.uk

Advice, support, training publications, magazine and insurance scheme. Links 16,000 community-based pre-schools.

For single parents
One Parent Families GINGERBREAD
255 Kentish Town Road
London NW5 2LX
Tel: 020 7428 5400
Lone parent helpline: 0800 018 5026 (weekdays 9am–5pm; Wed until 8pm)
Website: www.oneparentfamilies.org.uk

Free information leaflets and booklets, advice on benefits and rights, childcare and holidays. Can refer to other organisations who may be able to help.

Useful links
BBC Health Pages
Website: www.bbc.co.uk/health
Health pages from the BBC.

Patient UK
Website: www.patient.co.uk
A website with useful information about medical conditions for patients and health professionals.

The internet as a further source of information

After reading this book, you may feel that you would like further information on the subject. The internet is of course an excellent place to look and there are many websites with useful information about medical disorders, related charities and support groups.

For those who do not have a computer at home some bars and cafes offer facilities for accessing the internet. These are listed in the *Yellow Pages* under 'Internet Bars and Cafes' and 'Internet Providers'. Your local library offers a similar facility and has staff to help you find the information that you need.

It should always be remembered, however, that the internet is unregulated and anyone is free to set up a website and add information to it. Many websites offer impartial advice and information that has been compiled and checked by qualified medical professionals. Some, on the other hand, are run by commercial organisations with the purpose of promoting their own products. Others still are run by pressure groups, some of which will provide carefully assessed and accurate information whereas others may be suggesting medications or treatments that are not supported by the medical and scientific community.

Unless you know the address of the website you want to visit – for example, www.familydoctor.co.uk – you may find the following guidelines useful when searching the internet for information.

Search engines and other searchable sites

Google (www.google.co.uk) is the most popular search engine used in the UK, followed by Yahoo! (http://uk.yahoo.com) and MSN (www.msn.co.uk).

Also popular are the search engines provided by Internet Service Providers such as Tiscali and other sites such as the BBC site (www.bbc.co.uk).

In addition to the search engines that index the whole web, there are also medical sites with search facilities, which act almost like mini-search engines, but cover only medical topics or even a particular area of medicine. Again, it is wise to look at who is responsible for compiling the information offered to ensure that it is impartial and medically accurate. The NHS Direct site (www.nhsdirect. nhs.uk) is an example of a searchable medical site.

Links to many British medical charities can be found at the Association of Medical Research Charities' website (www.amrc.org.uk) and at Charity Choice (www.charitychoice.co.uk).

Search phrases

Be specific when entering a search phrase. Searching for information on 'cancer' will return results for many different types of cancer as well as on cancer in general. You may even find sites offering astrological information. More useful results will be returned by using search phrases such as 'lung cancer' and 'treatments for lung cancer'. Both Google and Yahoo! offer an advanced search option that includes the ability to search for the exact phrase, enclosing the search phrase in quotes, that is, 'treatments for lung cancer' will have the same effect. Limiting a search to an exact phrase reduces the number of results returned but it is best to refine a search to an exact match only if you are not getting useful results with a normal search. Adding 'UK' to your search term will bring up mainly British sites, so a good phrase might be 'lung cancer' UK (don't include UK within the quotes).

Always remember the internet is international and unregulated. It holds a wealth of valuable information but individual sites may be biased, out of date or just plain wrong. Family Doctor Publications accepts no responsibility for the content of links published in this series.

Index

Your pages

We have included the following pages because they may help you manage your illness or condition and its treatment.

Before an appointment with a health professional, it can be useful to write down a short list of questions of things that you do not understand, so that you can make sure that you do not forget anything.

Some of the sections may not be relevant to your circumstances.

We are always pleased to receive constructive criticism or suggestions about how to improve the books. You can contact us at:

Email: familydoctor@btinternet.com
Letter: Family Doctor Publications
PO Box 4664
Poole
BH15 1NN

Thank you

Health-care contact details

Name:

Job title:

Place of work:

Tel:

Name:

Job title:

Place of work:

Tel:

Name:

Job title:

Place of work:

Tel:

Name:

Job title:

Place of work:

Tel:

Significant past health events – illnesses/ operations/investigations/treatments

Event	Month	Year	Age (at time)

Appointments for health care

Name:

Place:

Date:

Time:

Tel:

Name:

Place:

Date:

Time:

Tel:

Name:

Place:

Date:

Time:

Tel:

Name:

Place:

Date:

Time:

Tel:

Appointments for health care

Name:

Place:

Date:

Time:

Tel:

Name:

Place:

Date:

Time:

Tel:

Name:

Place:

Date:

Time:

Tel:

Name:

Place:

Date:

Time:

Tel:

Current medication(s) prescribed by your doctor

Medicine name:

Purpose:

Frequency & dose:

Start date:

End date:

Medicine name:

Purpose:

Frequency & dose:

Start date:

End date:

Medicine name:

Purpose:

Frequency & dose:

Start date:

End date:

Medicine name:

Purpose:

Frequency & dose:

Start date:

End date:

Other medicines/supplements you are taking, not prescribed by your doctor

Medicine/treatment:

Purpose:

Frequency & dose:

Start date:

End date:

Medicine/treatment:

Purpose:

Frequency & dose:

Start date:

End date:

Medicine/treatment:

Purpose:

Frequency & dose:

Start date:

End date:

Medicine/treatment:

Purpose:

Frequency & dose:

Start date:

End date:

Questions to ask at appointments
(Note: do bear in mind that doctors work under great time pressure, so long lists may not be helpful for either of you)

Questions to ask at appointments
(Note: do bear in mind that doctors work under great time
pressure, so long lists may not be helpful for either of you)

Notes

Notes

Notes